T0324756

CONTROL AND THE THERAPEUTIC TRIAL

RHETORIC AND EXPERIMENTATION IN BRITAIN, 1918–48

THE WELLCOME SERIES
IN THE HISTORY OF MEDICINE

Forthcoming:

'A Cheap, Safe and Natural Medicine':
Religion, Medicine and Culture in John Wesley's Primitive Physic

Deborah Madden

The Wellcome Series in the History of Medicine series editors are
V. Nutton, M. Neve and R. Cooter.
Please send all queries regarding the series to Michael Laycock,
The Wellcome Trust Centre for the History of Medicine at UCL,
183 Euston Road, London NW1 2BE, UK.

CONTROL AND THE THERAPEUTIC TRIAL

RHETORIC AND EXPERIMENTATION IN BRITAIN, 1918–48

Martin Edwards

Amsterdam – New York, NY 2007

First published in 2007
by Editions Rodopi B. V., Amsterdam – New York, NY 2007.

Editions Rodopi B.V. © 2007

Design and Typesetting by Michael Laycock,
The Wellcome Trust Centre for the History of Medicine at UCL.
Printed and bound in The Netherlands by Editions Rodopi B.V.,
Amsterdam – New York, NY 2007.

Index by Liza Furnival.

British Library Cataloguing in Publication Data
A catalogue record for this book is available from the British Library

ISBN 978-90-420-2273-7

'Control and the Therapeutic Trial
Rhetoric and experimentation in Britain, 1918–48' –
Amsterdam – New York, NY:
Rodopi. – ill.
(Clio Medica 82 / ISSN 0045-7183;
The Wellcome Series in the History of Medicine)

Front cover:

A burning torch representing Hale's life tonic. Process print, *c.*1920.
Sir Ronald Ross, C.S. Sherrington, and R.W. Boyce in a laboratory at the Liverpool
School of Tropical Medicine. Gouache by W.T. Maud, 1899.
Images courtesy: Wellcome Library, London.

© Editions Rodopi B. V., Amsterdam – New York, NY 2007
Printed in The Netherlands

All titles in the Clio Medica series (from 1999 onwards) are available to
download from the IngentaConnect website: http://www.ingentaconnect.co.uk

Contents

Acknowledgements

Thanks to Professor Chris Lawrence for supervising the doctoral thesis from which this book derives. Thanks to Steve Sturdy and Tom Treasure for their suggestions and to Steve for his guidance regarding notions of control, also to the anonymous referee of my thesis for his/her useful comments. Thanks to everyone at The Wellcome Trust Centre for the History of Medicine at UCL for accepting me as part of their academic and social community; in particular I am grateful to Sally Bragg, Carmen Caballero-Navas, Caroline Essex, Emese Lafferton, Sharon Messenger, and Jane Seymour. I am indebted to all the friendly, efficient and ever-helpful staff both at The Wellcome Trust Centre and the Wellcome Library. I would also like to thank Harry Marks and Desiree Cox for their comments on parts of my original doctoral manuscript. A modified version of Chapter 2 has appeared as 'Good, Bad or Offal? The Evaluation of Raw Pancreas Therapy and the Rhetoric of Control in the Therapeutic Trial, 1925', *Annals of Science,* 61 (2004), 79–98, and is included here with permission from the publishers, Taylor and Francis (www.tandf.co.uk/journals).

I am grateful to The Health Foundation for a mid-career award grant which enabled me to carve out protected time to pursue these studies on a part-time basis, the Wellcome Trust for a research leave award, and to my colleagues in the Jenner Practice. Finally, I am eternally grateful to my wife Susan, for putting up with my devotion to the academic and social life of a medical historian when I should have been doing a proper job.

Note on National Archives Source Material

References such as 'FD1/5054' throughout this volume, refer to the cataloguing system in the British National Archives, where past documents of the MRC reside. The prefix 'FD' denotes MRC documentation.

Introduction

No word – as my next chapter proclaims – is innocent. Words carry implications, connotations, metaphorical associations, which are inherent and inescapable. Embedded within the phrase 'randomised controlled trial' (also in 'controlled trial', the Medical Research Council's preferred term up to the 1970s) is a word far from innocent; a powerful, dynamic, sexy, authoritative stormtrooper of a word. This is why I have chosen to write this history of rhetoric in the randomised controlled trial (RCT); existing histories of the RCT might be few in number, but some are nevertheless highly effective, as the following chapter will make clear. None, however, have chosen to examine the circumstances in which the term 'controlled' was employed in relation to therapeutic trials during the first half of the twentieth century, and the powerful rhetorical associations of the term – which, I shall argue, were exploited by the Medical Research Council (MRC) in its attempts to establish itself as the proper arbiter of therapeutic efficacy through experiment.

These arguments are developed in Chapter 1, 'No Word is Innocent: The Rhetoric of Controlled Trial Prior to 1948.' Here, I briefly summarise existing histories of therapeutic trials and the recent trend away from earlier, frequently present-centred and triumphalist narratives towards more critical analysis of therapeutic assessment within its social and historical context. I describe the variety of techniques to assess therapeutic efficacy which were available to a practitioner in early-twentieth-century Britain, and the MRC's attempts to establish itself and its own laboratory-orientated philosophy, as the proper channel for such investigation. I examine existing scholarship regarding the place of rhetoric in scientific discourse and attempt broadly to place the rhetoric of the MRC's use of the term 'controlled' within the context of therapeutic assessment.

This theme is examined in more detail in Chapter 2, 'Good, Bad or Offal? The Rhetoric of Control in the Evaluation of Raw Pancreas Therapy'. In 1925 a debate erupted in the correspondence columns of the *British Medical Journal* concerning the effectiveness of eating raw pancreas as a treatment for diabetes. Enthusiasts were predominantly general practitioners, who claimed success for the therapy on the basis of their clinical impressions. Their detractors were laboratory-orientated 'biochemist–physicians', who considered that their own experiments demonstrated that raw pancreas therapy was ineffective. The biochemist–physicians consistently dismissed the GPs' observations as inadequately 'controlled'. They did not define the meaning of 'controlled' in this context, although the biochemist–physicians' 'properly controlled' experiments involved careful regulation of their patients' diet and other environmental factors, and evaluation of the therapy's success through biochemical, rather than just clinical, criteria. However, these factors alone are inadequate to account for the biochemist–physicians' dismissal of the GPs' work as 'uncontrolled'. The biochemist–physicians were deliberately exploiting the powerful rhetorical connotations of the term 'control'. Ultimately, they implied that only a trial which they themselves had conducted, could be deemed 'adequately controlled'.

A similar analysis follows in Chapter 3, 'Bright Lights, Smoky Cities: Light Therapy in 1920s Britain.' MRC investigators found themselves on the back foot when their investigation of ultraviolet light therapy failed to establish the benefits of the technique for healing leg ulcers or for improving the health of weedy children. These negative findings attracted incredulity and opposition from medical professionals, whose consensus view almost universally supported the use of light therapy in the treatment of a wide variety of conditions. This was a broader and more public debate than that concerning the use of raw pancreas and saw MRC members on the defensive against general medical opinion – rather than on the offensive against a treatment favoured by a minority of (relatively low-status) practitioners, as in the raw pancreas debate. Nevertheless, the MRC again adopted the rhetoric of control in defence of its findings, arguing that they were valid because they were the product of 'controlled' work. The meaning of 'controlled' was, again, not defined but did not appear to refer solely to the presence of comparison subjects; rather, it performed further rhetorical functions.

A different issue of control arose when the MRC's newly-formed Therapeutic Trials Committee (TTC) inherited an ongoing MRC trial investigating the effectiveness of serum treatment for lobar pneumonia. In Chapter 4, 'Control and the MRC's Evaluation of Serum Therapy for Pneumonia, 1929–34,' I examine the serum therapy trial, and the TTC's criticisms when it assumed responsibility for the trial in 1931. The TTC deemed the trial's conduct, up to that point, unsatisfactory; the trial was even in danger of becoming an embarrassing source of humiliation for the MRC. The TTC imposed a number of new requirements on its researchers, including a unified plan of activity within the trial in future. Essentially the TTC attempted to impose centralised control over a set of investigators, some of whom it considered idiosyncratic, if not maverick, in their behaviour. The TTC was created expressly to undertake 'properly controlled clinical tests' of remedies; by bringing the serum trial under its central control, it rendered this trial 'controlled'. The notion of a 'controlled' trial, at this time, as one subject to centralised regulation is not new and a number of historians have described it. My analysis concerns the rhetorical function of the term 'controlled' and its implication of proper scrutiny and regulation.

By the 1940s, the ostensible meaning of the term 'controlled' had largely coalesced into a reference to the presence of a group of untreated comparison subjects within a therapeutic trial. However, the circumstances and contexts in which investigators chose actually to employ the term, exploited and emphasised its powerful rhetorical associations. In Chapter 5, 'Keeping it Controlled: The MRC's Trials of Immunisation against Influenza,' I examine a series of large-scale trials of influenza vaccine undertaken by the MRC immediately before, during, and immediately after the Second World War. The war rendered the search for an effective vaccine imperative, in view of the potentially devastating impact of any flu epidemic upon the combat capability of troops. The war and its aftermath also imposed particular difficulties upon the effective organisation of large-scale vaccine trials, notably due to scarce supplies of vaccine – which had, for the most part, to be imported from the United States or Commonwealth countries – and the mobility of populations, particularly fighting men and refugees. MRC workers frequently juxtaposed their use of the term 'controlled' alongside these difficulties. The MRC justified its monopoly over vaccine distribution by reference to the scarcity of supplies and the consequent need for vaccine distribution under the auspices of 'controlled trials'. With regard to unstable or mobile populations, the MRC again responded with reference to the need for 'controlled trials,' meaning trials which were organised and regulated by the MRC.

My sixth chapter, 'Whose Words are they Anyway? The Contrasting Strategies of Almroth Wright and Bradford Hill to Capture the Nomenclature of Controlled Trials,' examines the fundamental importance of nomenclature in forming notions of what a therapeutic trial was, the uses to which it could be put, and the questions that it was capable of answering. Austin Bradford Hill, commonly regarded as the chief originator of current RCT methodology, chose to employ words already in common use to explain trial methodology to a medical audience which possessed, on the whole, little statistical knowledge or interest. Almroth Wright, on the other hand, was a steadfast opponent of the 'statistical method' to ascertain therapeutic efficacy, preferring the certainty of laboratory experimentation followed by the judicious clinical impressions of an experienced physician. He considered 'statistical trials' to be useful only in a few particular circumstances. In common with his approach to other areas of scientific activity, he invented a series of new words to describe components of the statistical trial. By comparing Wright's invented words with those that Bradford Hill chose to describe equivalent concepts, I demonstrate that employing Wright's terminology results in a very different notion of the therapeutic trial, far more restricted in its scope and constrained in the uses to which it can be put, than a trial conceived under Bradford Hill's nomenclature.

In my conclusion, I examine some implications of this understanding of the rhetorical background to the development of the RCT, to current understanding and criticisms of therapeutic trials in particular, and to the broader debate around current attempts to promote evidence-based medicine. The rhetorical power of the term 'controlled' is still, I argue, very much a part of contemporary discourse concerning the persons and methods who should properly be charged with the assessment of therapeutic efficacy. It is possible that similar rhetorical capture is under way for other terms in the debate, notably 'evidence'.

1

No Word is Innocent:
The History and Rhetoric of Controlled Trials prior to 1948

Walter Morley Fletcher had only been in post as Secretary to the recently-formed Medical Research Committee for two years when, in 1916, he fell seriously ill with double pneumonia. He was dismayed to discover that his own physician's treatment, which included the application of leeches, was 'more worthy of the physicians of Charles the Second'.[1] Preferring a scientific remedy which was the product of recent research in a modern laboratory, he persuaded his friend Henry Dakin to let him have a supply of the new antiseptic chloramine. With the aid of a length of rubber tube from his dolls' house bath and the filling mechanism from a fountain pen, Fletcher administered the compound directly into his chest wound until he eventually recovered.

This experience can only have served to strengthen Fletcher's conviction that it was the laboratory, rather than the practising doctor, to which one should turn for the development and testing of new remedies, a conviction which profoundly influenced the philosophy of the Medical Research Committee and its successor the Medical Research Council (MRC) in the first half of the twentieth century. This chapter examines the role of the MRC in the early-twentieth-century debate over the proper means to evaluate the effectiveness of a remedy and, in particular, its use of the term 'controlled' as a rhetorical device to enhance its authority. This analysis is conducted against the background of existing historiography of the therapeutic trial, the state of therapeutic assessment during the first half of the twentieth century, and the relevance of rhetoric to scientific debate.

The MRC's streptomycin trial, published in 1948, provided a model for future work in studies of therapeutic efficacy. Prior to this, therapeutic trials were idiosyncratic affairs and the methodology of a proper clinical trial was neither unified nor codified. But the MRC nevertheless referred consistently to its own trials as 'controlled' throughout the first half of the twentieth century. The term encompassed an eclectic assortment of methodologies, and a number of different meanings were associated with it, sometimes simultaneously. Much of this volume is devoted to exploring these various meanings and the contexts in which they were used. The unifying characteristic which bound the divers uses of the term 'controlled', was its

9

use as a rhetorical device at a time when the authority to determine the proper means of testing a remedy was very much up for grabs. The MRC, by describing its own therapeutic experiments as 'controlled', was exploiting the powerful rhetorical connotations of the term. Ultimately, the MRC's 'controlled trial' became a construct – prior to 1948 there was no single methodology which could define the term, no published trial which could exemplify it, yet the 'controlled trial' was exploited as a rhetorical device to enhance the authority of a therapeutic experiment performed under the auspices of the MRC.

The randomised controlled trial in history

Nowadays, the proper means to assess the effectiveness of a new, or established, remedy is uncontroversial; the gold standard is the Randomised Controlled Trial (RCT). This involves comparing the clinical outcome of group of patients who receive the therapy under test, with an untreated control group. Frequently, the control group will receive a pharmacologically inert placebo (placebo control) and neither patients nor their physicians will be aware whether they are receiving active drug or placebo (double-blinding). Patients are allocated to receive active treatment or placebo strictly at random (randomisation.) According to Richard Smith, until recently editor of the *British Medical Journal,* the RCT could represent:

> [T]he most important development in medicine this [the twentieth] century… as important a change as that in the renaissance, when medicine began to base itself on experimental evidence rather than on reinterpreting the teachings of the ancients.[2]

By general consensus, the first published RCT was the MRC's trial of streptomycin in pulmonary tuberculosis in 1948. Its priority as the first RCT has been disputed; Sir Richard Doll[3] noted that the MRC designed and initiated its RCT of whooping cough vaccine before the streptomycin trial, although the whooping cough trial was published later. Others have accorded priority to earlier studies, for example Theobald's 1936 trial of vitamin supplementation in pregnancy toxaemia,[4] or Amberson's 1931 study of gold in the treatment of tuberculosis.[5] Nevertheless, the MRC presented its 1948 streptomycin trial as a new development at the time[6] and the trial subsequently represented a model – according to one commentator, a 'paradigm'[7] – for future therapeutic trials.

A number of historians have investigated the development of the RCT out of the eclectic collection of methodologies for drug evaluation available to an investigator during the early-twentieth century; others have chosen to trace the course of one specific component of RCT methodology, such as randomisation, blinding, or comparison groups. Some earlier histories of the controlled trial tend to be rather triumphalist narratives, implying a direct lineage for the RCT from Lind's naval trial of various scurvy remedies in 1747, or even earlier – Abraham Lilienfeld dates the use of comparison subjects in therapeutic assessment back to the biblical Book of Daniel,[8] and goes on to document sporadic use of comparisons including those by Petrarch in the fourteenth century. Other authors who assume this continuity narrative document a number of early clinical trials performed by those they consider forward-thinking pioneers, who adopted systematic methods of therapeutic research while their contemporaries were ignorant of the benefits. These pioneers variously include Avicenna, Celsus, Ambroise Paré's sixteenth-century comparison of battlefield wound treatments, Maitland's 1721 trial of smallpox inoculation on six convicts in Newgate prison, James Jurin's trial of smallpox inoculation in the 1720s, Lind's scurvy trial, William Withering's 1785 publication of his investigations into the foxglove, John Haygarth's use of placebo devices to denounce Perkin's skin tractors in 1801, Pierre Louis' 1837 trial of bloodletting in pneumonia, and Johannes Fibiger who in 1898 described the first use of allocation by alternation.[9]

These authors represent the failure of physicians en masse to adopt controlled trial methodology before the twentieth century as generally due to ignorance, the majority of practitioners choosing to disregard the example of their more enlightened colleagues who were attempting to pioneer the technique. Pocock[10] dismisses the 'subjective and extravagant claims' of eighteenth- and nineteenth-century researchers who he considers were insufficiently aware of the need for objective and statistically valid trials; John Prince Bull,[11] a physician working with the MRC Burns Unit during the 1940s and 1950s, dismisses ancient systems of medicine as irrational, ritualistic, or over-simplified; Shapiro and Shapiro[12] consider that ancient therapeutic assessment represented 'confusion and chaos'. Some commentators describe the increasing application of statistical methods to therapeutic research through the eighteenth and nineteenth centuries, until the development of the Chi-squared test by Pearson in 1900 and the t-test by Gosset – under the pseudonym 'Student' – in 1908, equipped investigators with probabilistic tools for statistical analysis.[13] The use of comparison controls increased through the 1920s and 1930s; randomisation is frequently attributed to the statistician Ronald Fisher, who first proposed it in 1923 as a statistical technique for investigating the yield of agricultural plots.[14] Austin Bradford Hill, apparently influenced by Fisher's work, applied randomisation to therapeutic investigation, culminating in the 1948 MRC streptomycin trial.

Aspects of this narrative have recently been questioned – particularly the reasons why pre-twentieth-century investigators did not adopt controlled trials, and the relevance of Fisher's statistical theory to Bradford Hill's incorporation of randomisation into therapeutic trials. Commentators have questioned the assumption that seventeenth- and eighteenth-century physicians ignored large-scale comparative trial methodology simply through ignorance, or missing the point. Tröhler,[15] Meldrum,[16] and Maehle[17] point out that such methodology was inappropriate to humoral medicine, whose remedies were uniquely tailored to an individual. 'Specifics' – remedies intended to treat a defined condition irrespective of the idiosyncracies of the recipient – were regarded with suspicion by most mainstream physicians, as the preserve of charlatans and quacks. Nineteenth- and twentieth-century physicians had their own reasons to be suspicious of numerical controlled trial methodology; in an influential account, Matthews[18] surveys the application of statistics to therapeutic assessment, and describes the scepticism expressed by clinicians, laboratory physiologists, and bacteriologists towards statistical methodology during the nineteenth and early-twentieth centuries. Statistical techniques represented an attempt to codify and quantify the making of medical knowledge, and were resisted by physicians who valued their professional autonomy and expertise. A number of other authors have described similar tensions between statistical methodology and clinicians' cherished bedside acumen.[19]

Matthews also credits Bradford Hill, the 'father of the modern clinical trial',[20] with applying statistics to therapeutic evaluation. However the origins of randomisation and Bradford Hill's reasons for adopting it, remain contentious. Ian Hacking[21] traces the origins of randomisation to experiments in psychology and psychic research during the late-nineteenth and early-twentieth centuries, some decades before its widespread adoption in therapeutic studies from the 1930s. Early experimenters in telepathy discovered that subjects would try to *guess* the next number, or next card, in a sequence that they were intended to receive telepathically from another subject. Presenting the numbers, or cards, in a random order prevented any such guessing strategies. Hacking suggests that these experiments could have influenced Fisher, who published a paper on card guessing in 1924, in his description of randomisation. Trudy Dehue[22] has extended this analysis, proposing that early-twentieth-century psychic research also promoted the use of randomly-allocated *groups* of comparison subjects, rather than simply randomisation of the order in which a subject received stimuli. She considers Fisher influential in the adoption of experimental randomisation, but points out that the technique was well established in these psychological circles before Fisher's advocacy. Many commentators agree that Bradford Hill was influenced by Fisher's statistical reasoning; Stephen Lock[23] credits Bradford Hill as the prime originator of the RCT and Fisher as the influence which led him to consider randomisation. The RCT was responsible for putting medicine on a rational scientific footing, he argues, and Bradford Hill was unfairly denied a Nobel Prize for establishing it.

Ted Kaptchuk[24] also attributes randomisation to Fisher, in an examination of the origins of blinding in therapeutic assessment. Blinding means that the patient (single-blind) or both patient and physician (double-blind) are unaware which preparation represents the therapy under test, and which the control. Kaptchuk traces a continuous two-hundred-year lineage for the use of blinding. Conventional physicians employed blinded assessment late in the eighteenth century to distinguish their remedies from those of unorthodox quacks, and the technique again came to prominence as a means to avoid fraud and the newly-described concept of 'suggestion' in psychological and psychic experiments during the late-nineteenth century. Experimenters employed placebos as an aid to blinding as early as 1834, when Trousseau tested a homeopathic remedy against inert bread pills, and was used in testing a mainstream remedy by Brown-Séquard in his 1889 comparison of injections of water and testicular extract. Kaptchuk argues that randomisation provided the impetus for blinding to become widely accepted in clinical trials from the 1930s onwards, despite initial resistance from many clinicians who considered that random allocation of subjects denied them their professional autonomy.

Recent scholarship has, however, questioned the relevance of Fisher's description of randomisation to its adoption in RCT methodology. Sir Iain Chalmers[25] questions notions of the RCT as a device invented by statisticians; he argues that statistical theory, including Fisher's advocacy of randomisation, had little influence on its development. Instead he represents the history of clinical trials as a history of attempts to reduce bias, culminating in the mid twentieth century when converging 'clinical' and 'statistical' reasons for adopting random allocation led to the development of the RCT. Chalmers regards Bradford Hill's experiences with the MRC's trial of serum therapy for pneumonia in the early-1930s as particularly formative, Hill realising that allocation of subjects by alternation[26] had allowed the introduction of bias which could be prevented by employing random allocation instead. My own analysis of the same trial, which follows in chapter 4 of this volume, supports Chalmers' conclusions. Benjamin Toth[27] also questions the influence of statisticians in general, and Bradford Hill in particular, on RCT design, instead presenting the use of statistics largely as a rhetorical device which enabled the MRC to represent its work as scientifically valid. He points out that randomised therapeutic trials were methodologically possible throughout the early-twentieth century, but considers that they were adopted only when randomisation suited the MRC's purposes by enabling it to exert a degree of control over the supply and use of streptomycin in the 1940s.

Recent investigations have also attempted to place twentieth-century therapeutic experimentation in social and historical context, situating the development of the RCT against a background of negotiations between physicians, laboratory scientists, government, the pharmaceutical industry, and the public. Toth[28] considers that the clinical trials organised by the MRC during the 1930s (some of which are explored later in this work) were 'historically inconsequential' as the MRC then prioritised laboratory methodology; the importance of these trials, he argues, was rather to consolidate the position of the MRC in relation to government, pharmaceutical companies, and the public. Alan Yoshioka[29] presents a similar argument with regard to the MRC's 1948 streptomycin trial and considers that the MRC adopted various strategies including emphasising the drug's toxicity, its scarcity, and the uncertainty over its efficacy, in order to establish its own control over supplies of the drug and over clinical trials in general.

Desiree Cox,[30] in her examination of the making of the clinical trial in Britain during the first half of the twentieth century, examines the MRC's attempts to establish itself as the arbiter of therapeutic efficacy and of drug standardisation. She describes Walter Fletcher's recruitment of 'noble scientists' – scientifically orientated physicians whom he considered to be trustworthy and of good character and who could reliably undertake therapeutic evaluation. The MRC established its Therapeutic Trials Committee (TTC) in 1931, intending it to run as a 'human machine,' a model of efficiency in drug evaluation; when the TTC was disbanded at the start of the Second World War, Cox argues, the clinical trial became mechanised into a mass event co-ordinated by statisticians. She presents the clinical trial as arising during the first four decades of the twentieth century as a co-ordinated system devised and performed by trustworthy characters, and points out that the procedural elements of the RCT were in place well before 1946. In the context of therapeutic reform in the United States, Harry Marks[31] similarly notes that RCT methodology had been available for years, indeed centuries, but only became generalised once the social and organisational means to pursue it, were in place. Early twentieth-century investigators had little infrastructure to support novel therapeutic research, and no exemplars of technique to follow. Marks charts the rise of laboratory-based 'rational therapeutics' late in the nineteenth century,[32] the transition of therapeutic investigation from a solitary to a co-operative venture, and twentieth-century calls for 'well controlled' therapeutic experiments which implied laboratory or quasi-laboratory hospital control of potentially confounding factors. Tragedies, such as deaths from contaminated sulfanilamide, and moral obligations highlighted by the Second World War, stimulated tighter central co-ordination of physicians' behaviour during therapeutic experimentation; Marks analyses the resultant negotiation of proper behaviour between physicians, drug companies, and government agencies. Randomisation and statistical analysis began to dominate trial methodology after 1950, largely, he argues, as the result of Bradford Hill's influence in Britain.

These recent analyses present the MRC as one party to a series of negotiations – with government, the pharmaceutical industry, the medical profession, and the public – over the proper means and the proper organisation or individuals, to conduct therapeutic research. I shall now turn to the environment in which a therapeutic investigator would work during the first half of the twentieth century, and the MRC's vigorous attempts, largely through the efforts of Walter Fletcher, to establish itself as the sole voice for medical research during this time.

Does it work?
The validation of therapeutic efficacy in the early-twentieth century

A physician practising in late-nineteenth or early-twentieth-century Britain was spoiled for choice from a large and rapidly expanding, selection of new and promising therapeutic options. During this 'golden age of medicine',[33] British physicians developed a renewed confidence regarding their understanding of disease and their ability effectively to treat it and an optimism that further spectacular advances were imminent. Generally attributed to the application of laboratory science in general, and germ theory in particular, the period saw the development of many new and powerful drugs. It also saw the appearance of a large number of therapies subsequently discredited as ineffective. Some were discredited shortly after their appearance; others not until they had been employed as remedies, sometimes extensively, for years or decades.

Some historians have chosen to document the appearance during this time, solely of those remedies which we would still regard as effective today. Ackerknecht[34] relates the discovery of vitamins, antibiotics, and later of steroid compounds, while Goodman chronicles therapeutic developments from the manufacture of the first synthetic antipyretic in 1883 through aspirin, diphtheria and tetanus antitoxins, Salvarsan, Prontosil, vitamins, and hormones, and concludes that 'Vitamins, hormones, insulin and the sulfa drugs were the great therapeutic successes of the inter-war period.'[35] Brandt and Gardner[36] point to the development of the antibacterial 'magic bullets' Salvarsan, Prontosil (sulfanilamide), penicillin, and streptomycin during the first half of the twentieth century. However, there is an internalist approach implicit in ignoring the considerable number of treatments which were subsequently abandoned as ineffective, which also appeared during this time. Guenter Risse[37] has surveyed the 'Whiggish' nature of many histories of therapeutics, which he claims tend to dismiss as inexplicable 'fads'

15

practitioners' use of remedies which we would now deem ineffective. Risse concludes with a plea that therapies should be analysed with a view to the social context in which they were employed. Certainly many 'ineffective' remedies were enthusiastically adopted in the first half of the twentieth century, for years or decades, by a large proportion, even a majority, of practitioners, who were convinced of their effectiveness and who saw a great and sustained future ahead for them. Later in this work I shall explore some examples – raw pancreas therapy for diabetes in 1925, ultra-violet light therapy in the late-1920s, and serum treatment for pneumonia in the 1930s. Lawrence[38] points to further instances – therapeutic vaccines, tuberculin treatment for tuberculosis, and the myriad varieties of glandular therapy popular in the 1920s and 1930s. Any retrospective attempt to examine 'effective' therapies in isolation from those we now deem 'ineffective' misses the point, that our current notions of a treatment's merits or otherwise were not apparent to physicians at the time. Whether a treatment 'works' is a socially and culturally bound conclusion,[39] and can be fiendishly difficult for a practising clinician to assess. New therapies were widespread during the first half of the twentieth century, each held its own promise and had its own advocates, and each required some form of verification. How was a practitioner to assess the effectiveness of a remedy? In fact, our practitioner was spoiled for choice – together with the rise in the number of available therapies, a variety of methodologies, both novel and established, was available with which to judge their efficacy.

Prior to the First World War, therapeutic research in the UK was largely an individual affair, practised by 'enthusiastic clinicians in their spare time'.[40] Medical reformers sought to increase the influence of science in therapeutics, particularly through the formation of university departments of medicine. The Haldane Commission, which reported on the workings of the London teaching hospitals in 1913, provided a major impetus to the establishment of such professorial units.[41] Six units were established in the UK by 1921, and thirteen by 1944, largely as the result of benefactions from the Rockefeller Foundation in the US which provided direct capital funding for a number of units, freeing UK government spending for recurrent costs.[42] These units largely promoted a laboratory-orientated concept of science in their clinical investigations. Christopher Lawrence[43] described how clinical researchers during the inter-war years, influenced by these professorial units, adopted an increasing division of labour. As clinicians attempted to co-ordinate large scale co-operative studies, their therapeutic investigations became typified by teamwork, rather than individual endeavour. Harry Marks[44] provides a similar analysis in his description of US therapeutic reform. He described the transition from therapeutic research conducted by individuals, early in the twentieth century, through larger co-operative studies intended to pool the experience of many physicians, to the establishment of the Randomised Controlled Trial in the second half of the century.

The first half of the twentieth century therefore offered a variety of methods to a practitioner attempting to ascertain the efficacy of a new therapeutic agent and accounts of therapeutic investigations in contemporary medical journals reflected this diversity. Traditional case reports detailing a single practitioner's experience with a therapy given to one or more patients had been the standard vehicle for transmitting conclusions regarding a therapy's worth since the Renaissance, and remained commonplace. Laboratory studies involving animals, humans, or *in vitro* pathology specimens, were frequently reported. Larger therapeutic trials, in which a clinician – or a team of clinicians and scientists – administered treatment to a group of patients, frequently aggregating the results by some means such as a table or by calculating an average, became more prevalent during the 1920s and 1930s. A minority of such studies employed an untreated comparison group.

Notions of the therapeutic trial reflected this spectrum of opinion. To some, a properly conducted trial represented a quantitative study of the physiological effects of a drug upon animals or human volunteers in a laboratory.[45] To others, it represented careful scrutiny of the clinical effects of a therapy administered in the environmentally regulated conditions of a teaching hospital, frequently to selected groups of patients.[46] To the remainder, the observation of individual patients treated in private, hospital or domestic practice was superior, backed up as it was by the physician's experience and expertise;[47] these findings would generally be presented as case reports, from which the clinician would derive his conclusions. Not infrequently, different methodologies for assessing a treatment's worth would produce conflicting results, and two particular examples – concerning the therapeutic value of raw pancreas, and of ultra-violet light – are explored in this work. As will become apparent from these later chapters, clinicians often argued vehemently for the value of their own chosen methodology, and of the conclusions they drew from it regarding a therapy's value. The stakes in the debate were high, involving no less than the moral authority to adjudicate on the effectiveness of medical therapy. Unsurprisingly, the protagonists employed a variety of debating strategies to promote their own cause.

The MRC and therapeutic efficacy

The Medical Research Council was a major player in this arena and much of my argument concerns the rhetorical strategies which it employed, during the first half of the twentieth century, to establish itself and its methodologies as the proper arbiters of therapeutic efficacy. The MRC arose as a continuation of the Medical Research Committee, created by the government in 1913, and re-established as the Medical Research Council in 1920 in order to avoid its subjugation to the newly-created Ministry of Health.[48] Walter Morley Fletcher (1873–1933) was its Secretary from 1914 until his death in 1933, and exerted an immense influence on the MRC's philosophy and activity.[49] Until Fletcher's appointment, the Committee had operated along the lines of a gentleman's dining club, meeting in the home of its chairman, Lord Moulton, and seemingly 'running around in circles for a year, enjoying Lord Moulton's excellent dinners and wit'[50] until Fletcher took it in hand.

Fletcher was working in Michael Foster's school of physiology in Cambridge when he was offered the post of Secretary to the Medical Research Committee. A keen athlete during his undergraduate years at Trinity College Cambridge, he took his BA in Natural Sciences in 1894 and proceeded to work in physiological studies, becoming a Fellow of Trinity in 1897. Choosing to add a medical degree to his qualifications he won a scholarship to St Bartholomew's Hospital and gained his MB in 1900, returning again to Cambridge where he was a Fellow and lecturer, and from 1904 to 1914 a tutor, at Trinity College. He gained his MD in 1908 and was elected FRS in 1915 as a result of his work with Gowland Hopkins on muscle metabolism. He was knighted in 1918. His influence on the philosophy of the MRC and indeed on the direction of medical research in Britain, was immense. Quick-tempered at times, and not given to suffering fools gladly, he nevertheless gained the reputation of fierce ally once a worker had gained his confidence.[51]

From his appointment as secretary to the Medical Research Committee in 1914, Fletcher consistently prioritised basic biomedical science and a laboratory-based epistemology. He repeatedly affirmed his conviction that medicine and therapeutics could only progress through fundamental scientific research, frequently performed by non-clinical scientists rather than clinicians. In particular, he apparently did not consider that GPs had a great deal, or indeed anything, to contribute to this endeavour.[52] He was equally fervent in his belief that medical research in Britain should be controlled exclusively by the MRC. Joan Austoker[53] documents his efforts to discourage, right from the outset, any attempts to organise medical research outside his own sphere of influence, including his conflict with the Imperial Cancer Research Fund (ICRF) in 1918 and competition with the Ministry of Health over the right to perform clinical research. Fletcher fought vigorously and successfully to prevent the MRC becoming incorporated into the newly formed Ministry of Health following the First World War, arguing forcibly for the 'scientific independence of medical research.'[54] Several years of spats with the Ministry ensued until Fletcher finally agreed a 'concordat' with George Newman, the Minister of Health, with whom Fletcher rarely saw eye-to-eye, in 1924. This agreement defined the respective activities of the MRC and Ministry of Health, and allowed the MRC a wide reign over biomedical research,[55] besides forming a principal conduit for research income from the Rockefeller and Dunn research funds.

Fletcher's relationship with the British Empire Cancer Campaign (BECC), formed in 1923 to help fund and organise cancer research, was also acrimonious[56] – his response upon hearing of the new organisation was 'to remind you that the Medical Research Council is the body specially charged by the Government and Parliament with the duty of supporting and encouraging work in *all* branches of medicine.'[57] His opposition to the BECC bought him into direct conflict with some of the most eminent physicians and surgeons of the day, including Sir John Bland-Sutton, Sir Charles Gordon Watson, Sir Bernard Spilsbury, and J.P. Lockhart-Mummery, who were among the BECC's founder members. Lord Horder, another founder, bitterly criticised Fletcher for his 'activities in the direction of monopolising and controlling medical research.'[58] Fletcher argued that clinicians were essentially useless in co-ordinating cancer research,[59] which he said should be under the control of MRC scientists. He continued to clash with the clinical elite throughout the subsequent decade, when he opposed attempts by the Royal Colleges to exert control over clinical and therapeutic research. Austoker[60] and Rosemary Stevens[61] both describe how the MRC, with its support for a new breed of scientifically-orientated, specialist clinical practitioner, was viewed with suspicion by the Colleges which sought to maintain their own autonomy and control over a profession which they preferred to view as unified, not divided by specialisation. Fletcher was equally unimpressed by the Colleges; David Cantor,[62] in an examination of the conflict between the Colleges and the MRC over access to and use of radium in the inter-war years, concludes that Fletcher adopted three specific strategies – controlling the membership of the BECC Committee; moving research away from elite London hospitals; and encouraging co-operation between clinicians and scientists – to fend off 'practitioner control of scientific research.'

Claiming in 1930 to speak on behalf of the Royal Colleges, Sir Berkeley (later Lord) Moynihan, President of the Royal College of Surgeons, expressed resentment of the MRC's 'disdain' for clinicians and their clinical activity.[63] Fletcher's response was characteristically robust, emphasising the importance of fundamental biomedical investigation and pointing out clinicians' inability to manage research in a competent fashion.[64] In 1932, the availability of Leverhulme funds enabled the Royal College of Physicians (RCP) to contemplate the creation of its own programme of clinical research; Fletcher, in declining health during what was to be the last year of his life, vigorously opposed what he perceived as a threat to the MRC's control. Lord Dawson, the RCP president, criticised the MRC for adopting a superior, 'highbrow' stance over 'lowbrow' clinicians and enquired whether medicine was really so inefficient that it needed the MRC to do its research; Fletcher's blunt response was in the affirmative.[65] The argument even became the subject of lay criticism, the *Daily Herald* complaining that research funds were being wasted through jealousy between 'doctors and scientists' as the debate raged on.[66]

In their spat with the MRC, the Royal Colleges were defending their members' clinical autonomy and the virtues of incommunicable wisdom and clinical expertise in assessing clinical outcomes, against the MRC's laboratory-orientated epistemology. This represented one of a number of disputes between 'doctors and scientists' in the early-twentieth century, some of which have formed the subject of recent scholarship. Christopher Lawrence has characterised the tensions between elite 'patrician' practitioners and the newer breed of laboratory-orientated physicians during the early-twentieth century.[67] Describing the increasing application of laboratory science to clinical medicine, Lawrence argues that enthusiasts for laboratory techniques were countered by 'patrician' clinicians who valued individual bedside clinical acumen which, they said, could only arise from broad learning, proper upbringing, and extensive clinical experience. Individual practitioners frequently occupied positions along a spectrum of views between these two extremes, such as the clinician and MRC investigator John Ryle, whose contribution to one MRC study is documented in a later chapter concerning the MRC's trial of serum therapy. In an analysis of parallel tensions between clinicians and scientists in the United States, Gerald Geison documents the development of physiology as an independent discipline by the beginning of the twentieth century and its mutually-dependent relationship with clinical medicine – physiologists were dependent on clinical medicine for their funding and validity, but clinical medicine relied upon physiology to verify its credentials as a scientific discipline.[68] Clinicians remained sceptical of the value of physiology; Steve Sturdy describes the MRC's less than entirely successful attempts to promote the results of oxygen therapy as a triumph for the physiological method during the First World War.[69] Russell Maulitz similarly examines tensions between American bacteriologists and clinicians, whose attempts to assimilate the scientific legitimacy of bacteriology led to redefinitions of the meaning of 'science' within clinical medicine.[70] Laboratory pharmacologists also clashed with their clinical colleagues over the value and proper place of their discipline. John Parascandola describes the debate between pharmacologists, notably Henry Dale, and clinicians over the value of ergot in obstetric practice; ultimately a resolution was only achieved by co-operative investigation involving both disciplines.[71] Laboratory science's ultimate success in incorporating itself within the fabric of clinical medicine was not due to its self-evident superiority, indeed, Geison acknowledges that its opponents were largely correct in discounting it as irrelevant to clinical practice.[72] Rather, Steve Sturdy and Roger Cooter suggest that laboratory-based science partly owed its ascendancy to the nature of its organisation, featuring salaried clinicians in a large administrative structure employing teamwork, which accorded with the increasingly corporate nature of mass health care in the first half of the twentieth century.[73]

Fletcher numbered himself firmly with the scientists in this dispute and remained tireless in his advocacy of the MRC as the only proper authority to co-ordinate and control clinical research in Britain. Much of the remainder of this volume examines some of the rhetorical strategies which he and his MRC allies adopted to defend this claim. Fletcher definitely included the proper means to determine therapeutic efficacy as being within this sphere of MRC control; from its inception, the MRC was involved in assessing the worth of remedies, portraying itself as an authoritative and independent arbiter of therapeutic effectiveness and drug quality. Jonathan Liebenau[74] and Desiree Cox[75] describe the MRC's involvement in the standardisation and regulation of new drugs, from its role in testing the quality of British-manufactured Salvarsan in 1916 – German supplies having been interrupted by the war – to its petitioning the Government the following year to be allowed to regulate all manner of other new preparations including sera and vaccines. The MRC obtained unique control of scarce supplies of insulin for clinical trials in 1922, streptomycin in 1946, and attempted to exert similar control over supplies of radium between 1920 and 1939.[76] The MRC provided financial and moral support for a number of other therapeutic trials performed by individuals it regarded as trustworthy – the 'noble scientists' of Cox's analysis.[77] So important did the evaluation of therapeutic efficacy become to the MRC that in 1931 it established its own Therapeutic Trials Committee (TTC) specifically to assess the merits of new remedies. The demand for therapeutic trials had expanded, party due to the increasing number of new preparations which were appearing and which were largely created by British drug manufacturers who sought a means of validating their remedies comparable to the system which existed in Germany. There, individual physicians would assess and personally endorse a new remedy; British doctors, however, were generally reluctant to associate themselves with the verification of a drug's efficacy for fear of being accused of having an inappropriate pecuniary interest.[78] The MRC, therefore, decided to create 'a more regular machinery for the organisation of clinical trials'[79] and announced the creation of the TTC, which would arrange 'properly controlled clinical tests of new products.'[80]

Cox[81] points out that prior to the establishment of the TTC, the MRC would generally send samples of a new drug to investigators at different centres, each of whom would test it in his own idiosyncratic way. Insulin, for example, was variously tested by administering it to normal and diabetic subjects and measuring their blood glucose and weight gain, by administering it to diabetics and observing the clinical effects, or by attempting to standardise the insulin requirements of different individuals – all at the whim of the investigator, although the MRC did require the investigating team invariably to include a biochemist. These insulin trials served as a paradigm for subsequent investigations, for example of liver extract in pernicious anaemia, sanocrysin, and 'diaplyte vaccine', all tested according to the personal inclinations of individual physicians. Cox[82] suggests that the ongoing trial of serum therapy for pneumonia which the TTC inherited at its inception – and which I discuss later in this work – established a model and a set of methodological guidelines, for future trials, including the use of untreated comparison subjects and allocation of subjects to the treated or untreated group by alternation. Landsborough Thomson makes a similar claim, arguing that by the time it was disbanded the TTC had 'set a standard for the methods of trial...'[83] Other historians appear to have reproduced this claim rather uncritically; for example Meldrum follows Landsborough Thomson, and credits the TTC with codifying techniques such as randomisation and blinding into a methodology.[84] However, I would argue that the MRC's attempts to present the output of the TTC as representative of a unified therapeutic trial methodology were essentially rhetorical. Examination of the trials published by the TTC until its winding-up at the start of the Second World War, rather belies any suggestion that a unified methodology was in place.[85] A minority of studies employed untreated or placebo-treated[86] comparison subjects, sometimes referred to as 'controls'.[87] Subjects in these studies were allocated to receive active or inactive therapy either by alternation[88] or at the discretion of the investigator, who frequently allotted most of his patients to receive the new drug, reserving just a few as 'controls'.[89] A few compared the effect of two or more different drugs without any untreated subjects,[90] or administered both active and inactive drugs to all patients at different times – the inactive preparation, rather than the subject, forming the 'control'.[91] Many more trials were simply case reports, describing the effects of drug therapy on any number of patients from one,[92] to a handful,[93] or a series of a hundred or more.[94] Most authors simply described these case reports in some narrative detail;[95] others presented additional animal experiments[96] or employed detailed quantification and tabulation of findings such as blood pressure, blood chemistry, weight, temperature, signs and symptoms.[97]

The extent to which the TTC even *could* have imposed a unified methodology upon its workers, had it possessed one, is also questionable. Many of the investigators cherished their autonomy and disliked being dictated to (see Chapter 4 in this volume on serum therapy) and Toth[98] points out that the TTC, with no clinical facilities of its own, was entirely dependent on its investigators' goodwill for access to patients. Toth[99] also describes the rise in British drug companies' confidence and assertiveness during the life of the TTC and their increasing ability to dictate terms to the Committee. He concludes that, as a result, the TTC did not introduce any methodological innovation during its existence.[100] Nonetheless, as Cox[101] has effectively argued, the MRC did represent its TTC as an efficient, and uniquely British, machine for evaluating new drugs. I suggest that this presentation was largely a rhetorical device to help establish the authority of the MRC in the arena of therapeutic evaluation.

No word is innocent:
Rhetoric and the therapeutic evaluation debate

Recently, some historians have chosen to highlight the importance to the MRC of presentation and rhetoric during its attempts, throughout the first half of the twentieth century, to establish itself as the sole proper arbiter of therapeutic efficacy. Toth, in playing down the importance of statistical theory in the creation of the RCT, represents the MRC's claims to employ statistics as a rhetorical device. 'Statistics [in this context] are rhetoric; they are verbal tactics deployed to create epistemological and practical advantage'.[102] Yoshioka[103] also examines the importance of presentation and emphasis in the MRC's 1948 streptomycin trial, arguing that the MRC exaggerated the scarcity and toxicity of the drug and the uncertainty over its effectiveness in order to secure control over its distribution. Cox describes the importance of presentation to Fletcher himself, suggesting that the clinical trial under his direction was a deliberately 'invented tradition'[104] and that Fletcher chose to present himself in a particular light, playing up his associations with Trinity College Cambridge and inventing a Cambridge history.[105] Cantor highlights the importance to protagonists in the 1920s debate between surgeons and the MRC over access to supplies of radium for research, of establishing the right to adopt the rhetoric of science as their own.[106] Meldrum represents the RCT itself as a social construct, one important function of which is essentially rhetorical, in validating researchers' claims for scientific objectivity.[107]

The notion that rhetoric is inherent in even the most technical scientific or medical accounts, is well established. This view regards rhetoric as a fundamental, inseparable component of discourse and not as an empty or devious device with the adverse connotations which John Schuster and Richard Yeo describe as 'mere rhetoric, in the traditional perjorative sense of rhetoric as a mere art of persuasion.'[108] Rather, they argue, rhetoric is an inherent part of the complex process of producing and ratifying scientific knowledge.[109] Yeo[110] regards scientific activity as essentially a process of negotiation, to which rhetoric is fundamental. Marcello Pera defines scientific rhetoric as 'the art of making use of persuasive arguments in order to change or reinforce opinions in a scientific community,'[111] and discusses its implicit use in the writings of scientists including Galileo and Darwin. Scientific language, these authors argue, cannot be considered 'objective' or be stripped of its – frequently powerful – rhetorical and metaphorical associations. Jan Golinski[112] considers that scientific terms inevitably carry metaphorical associations which may differ from one individual to the next, and argues that capturing the vocabulary in a debate can render the other side powerless, without a means to express its ideas – as was the case with Lavoisier's chemical nomenclature.[113] Philip Kitcher[114] also regards rhetoric as 'inescapable'[115] in any scientific discourse, including even mathematical statements, and analyses examples of embedded rhetoric in Darwin's writings. Similarly, Charles Bazerman's[116] studies of scientific writings from 1665 to the twentieth century establish the presence of an inherent rhetorical, persuasive function of language, although Bazerman argues that scientists themselves are generally unaware of these unconscious rhetorical devices.[117] Scott Montgomery[118] also traces inherent rhetoric in scientific writing by Chaucer, Bacon, Galileo, Boyle, and Newton and analyses scientific writings up to the late-twentieth century. He describes changes in style – a trend towards more simplified accounts during the early-twentieth century, for example – but with presentational techniques and rhetoric interwoven throughout.

This analysis of rhetorical effect, conscious or otherwise, applies equally to the nuances of individual words; as Montgomery warns, 'No word is innocent... language, after all, cannot be deprived of its *meaningful* connotative associations and urges; frames of reference always leak.'[119] Individual words inevitably convey metaphorical associations, indeed, commentators such as George Lakoff and Mark Johnson[120] argue that the human conceptual system is fundamentally metaphorical in nature and that such metaphorical associations are not merely inescapable, they are a constituent part of thought and communication. But the meanings of words, their historical and social connotations, and their relationships with other words can change with time, a notion which Raymond Williams[121] cites as a central justification for his analysis of 'keywords' in the English language. Accordingly, a few individual words or terms in the history of science, have formed the object of sustained study. Robert Young[122] has examined Darwin's use of the terms 'selection' and 'natural selection', describing how Darwin modified his use of the terms as he modified his theories but nevertheless self-consciously continued to employ them despite opposition from others such as Wallace and Lyell because of their rhetorical appeal to a wider, non-scientific audience. Young explicitly defends his decision to examine a single metaphor 'in isolation', arguing that the term 'natural selection' represents the central explanatory principle of Darwin's writing and is 'anthropomorphic, deeply ambiguous, and amenable to all sorts of readings and modifications.'[123] Roger Smith[124] has examined the changing meanings and usage of the word 'inhibition' in neurophysiology and psychology from the nineteenth to mid-twentieth centuries, embedding the use of the term in changing Victorian and twentieth-century social values. He, too, defends his examination of a single word, arguing that the non-technical uses of a word cannot be divorced from its other connotations.[125] Christopher Lawrence has performed a similar analysis of Lister's use of the word 'putrefaction',[126] arguing that Lister initially employed the term to represent a process akin to fermentation but changed the meaning he attributed to it a number of times in order, retrospectively, to align his theories with ascendent German germ theory during the 1880s.

'Control' in early-twentieth-century Britain

This volume is similarly devoted largely to the examination of a single word – 'controlled' – in the context of the rhetoric of the debate over therapeutic evaluation between 1918 and 1948. The word is a powerful one, with powerful associations.[127] To be 'controlled' or 'under control' implies that everything is in order; to be 'uncontrolled' or 'out of control' implies dangerous disorder. 'Controlled' may carry associations of subjugation, overpowering, domination, or command, and implications of authority and power. Unsurprisingly, the MRC sought to adopt it – and its potent rhetorical associations – to describe its own studies in therapeutic evaluation. The term has received little analysis from historians to date, although Smith[128] discusses it as a significant component of some of the meanings of 'inhibition'. He emphasises the importance of 'control' to Victorian society, which he presents as a lifelong struggle for moral control to enable an individual to lead a good life. Control of individuals by others, control of groups and individuals within society, control of women by men, and control of sexual desire and masturbation formed important components of Victorian notions of control, with deviant behaviour, drunkenness, and mental illness forming a stark reminder of the dire effects of loss of control.

Notions of control acquired fresh associations – with ordered, scientific activity besides proper moral behaviour – in early-twentieth-century British society, with the influx of American thinking on scientific management and engineering process. Frederick Taylor (1856–1915) attempted to improve the efficiency and productivity of industrial working practices by redesigning them along 'scientific' lines.[129] Time-and-motion studies allowed the fragmentation of workers' activity into a series of standardised tasks to be adopted by all workers. The system imposed control over workers, by designating them a specific sequence of activity from which they must not deviate and also required that they be subject to surveillance to ensure that they were performing as expected. This latter requirement was facilitated by the rise in feedback control in industrial and other engineering processes – a major new industry in industrial indicators, recorders and controllers arose from the 1920s, and by the 1930s, 'controllers' constituted around half of all new industrial instruments offered for sale. Stuart Bennett[130] has pointed out that these devices were actually employed largely as a means of surveillance by management over the activity of their workforce, and frequently they were located in the manager's office or a central control room rather than anywhere the workers could read them. Such instruments enabled employers to impose quasi-laboratory conditions in the workplace, controlling workers' performance and the physical environment. The instruments offered information which would hitherto have remained part of the 'art and mystery' of a craft, demystifying workers' activities, and leaving the workforce open to the imposition of scientific management.

The scientific efficiency movement impinged upon medicine too; in the United States, the American College of Surgeons appropriated initiatives to restructure hospital practice along Taylorist principles in order successfully to control inter-war hospital organisation.[131] Even the reorganisation and standardisation of medical records in the name of scientific practice, shifted relationships of power and control within hospitals.[132] In medicine as well as industry, the rhetoric of scientific method and scientific practice had become increasingly conflated with that of control. This resonates with contemporary notions of 'control' in therapeutic trials, where, as we shall see, the term was used *inter alia* to imply scrutiny, efficiency, and proper organisation of participants' behaviour.

Within biological science, notions of control from the mid-nineteenth century generally implied accurate regulation of the internal and external physical environment of an organism within a laboratory experiment. The nineteenth-century shift from vitalist to mechanistic concepts of life processes had opened up such functions for investigation by experiment and by machines, such as the calorimeter. Claude Bernard emphasised the importance of such experimental control from 1850, stressing the need for 'control over all conditions affecting the organism' before the physiologist could do his work.[133] A properly controlled experiment was therefore one which maintained a constant physiological environment – 'control' here implying 'restraint' – whilst allowing the experimenter to vary the independent variable – here 'control' implies 'guidance'.[134] From the end of the nineteenth century, an additional usage of the term 'control' appeared within biological experimentation; control as a check, a comparison against which to judge the outcome of an intervention. This remains the current mainstream technical meaning of the term; the outcome of an experimental manipulation – for example, administration of a drug – is checked against the outcome amongst subject(s) who have not received the intervention, to confirm that the intervention is indeed the cause of any observed change. Edwin Boring has pointed out that the very origins of the term 'control' – which derives from *contre-roll* or counter-roll, a duplicate accounting register against which the original could be verified – imply this use as a check. From the 1870s, he traces instances of 'control' used in this way, from Darwin's 1875 description of a 'control experiment' in relation to the way plant bladders react to food, to Hankin's 1890 *Nature* article in which his use of the term 'control mice' without further explanation implies that this usage is by this time widely accepted. Control *groups* – where an entire set of untreated or unmanipulated subjects was used for comparison – first arose from learning transfer experiments in the early-twentieth century.[135] Effective statistical techniques for comparing data between different groups began to appear at the same time – Pearson first described the chi-squared test in 1900 and William Gosset published the t-test under the pseudonym 'Student' in 1908 – but these probably co-incided with the employment of control groups rather than inspiring their use.[136]

Nowadays, the technical meaning of the term 'controlled' in the context of a therapeutic trial is uncontroversial – it refers to the presence of an untreated, or differently-treated, 'control' group of patients whose outcome can be compared with the group receiving the treatment under test. This 'technical' term is nevertheless still redolent with rhetorical associations, as the following chapters should demonstrate. This technical meaning appears to have coalesced during the late-1930s and 1940s and to have hardened following the MRC's adoption of its 1948 streptomycin trial as an exemplar. Throughout the first half of the twentieth century, however, the term had no single technical meaning, nor was any concerted attempt made to define one. I consider that this allowed the MRC to exploit the metaphorical associations of this rhetorically powerful, but loosely defined, word. Until the mid-twentieth century, the MRC did not use the term 'controlled' to imply a particular methodology; I have already alluded to the diversity of techniques which the MRC's investigators chose to employ when investigating the efficacy of new remedies during this time. Nevertheless, the MRC chose to represent its own trials under the rubric 'controlled'. The announcement of the formation of the TTC promised 'properly controlled clinical tests of new products'[137] and the term 'controlled' repeatedly appeared in MRC investigators' descriptions of their own work – particularly, as subsequent chapters will demonstrate, when defending their findings or attacking those of others. Some historians have commented upon the looseness with which the term was applied and have attempted to infer a number of different meanings of 'controlled' according to the context in which it was used – meanings which extend well beyond the notions of controls as restraint, guidance, or a check initially described by Boring. Toth considers that:

> The meaning of the word control varied considerably among those who used it. The only shared feature was the connotation that by controlling their results something precise and scientific was being offered.[138]

Marks[139] points to a variety of understandings of the term 'controlled' in the United States, incorporating untreated comparison subjects, well-planned experiments, or careful scrutiny and regulation of the patients' environment which almost inevitably implied a hospital setting. Cox,[140] in her analysis of the MRC's serum therapy trial (see Chapter 5 of this volume) also concludes that the physicians involved interpreted the ideals of a 'controlled experiment' in a number of different, idiosyncratic ways – including close clinical scrutiny and recording of cases, comparison with an untreated group, comparison with a group of patients receiving different active therapy, and regulation of the patients' environment within the hospital ward. Other implicit meanings of the term which appear throughout the 1920s and 1930s include the use of laboratory analysis rather than clinical observation to assess the outcome of cases,[141] and strict scrutiny and regulation of factors in the patients' environment such as diet, exercise, nursing care, and even their dosage of laxatives and daily exposure to sunlight.[142] The increasing MRC exploitation of the term did not escape satirical attention; in 1943 a *Daily Mail* reporter attempted to procure treatment with patulin, a penicillin derivative which had gained popular acclaim as a wonder cure for the common cold, and which was the subject of an MRC 'controlled' trial.

> I suggested that I was recovering from a streaming cold and might prove an acceptable human guinea pig for experiment' suggested the reporter, 'but the answer was again 'no,' I was not 'controlled' any more than the hundred others who had applied by telephone during the morning.[143]

The unfortunate reporter had encountered a further use of the term 'controlled', considered in more detail in the later chapter in this volume concerning influenza vaccination; as a device to regulate supply of a scarce drug.

Much of the remainder of this volume is devoted to exploring the contexts in which MRC workers employed the term 'controlled', and the meanings they ascribed to it. Ultimately, I shall argue, the word represented more than the sum of its parts. It was not simply an innocent word with a number of distinct technical meanings; no word is innocent. The contexts in which MRC workers chose to use 'controlled' cannot entirely be explained by examining its various technical meanings. Rather, the term became employed as a rhetorical device to help the MRC secure its position as the only proper arbiter of therapeutic efficacy. Cox alludes to such a notion in her description of the influence of statisticians upon clinical trials during the 1930s:

> Physicians involved in trials took the idea of dividing the patients into control and treatment groups as a given, using 'controls' and alternating groups more as a rhetorical stick than a category with a universal meaning. Thus, it is not so much the issue of where these ideas may have come from which informs us about the making of the clinical trial, but the question of who claimed these tools for the specific purpose of medical research.[144]

Those employing the term 'controlled' as a rhetorical tool on behalf of the MRC were the laboratory-orientated, statistically-minded physician–scientists who were held in such high regard by Fletcher. The term increasingly became associated with statisticians during the 1940s, but we shall now trace its use, and the influence of its rhetorical connotations, from the early-1920s.

Notes

1. M. Fletcher, *The Bright Countenance: A Personal Biography of Walter Morley Fletcher* (London: Hodder and Stoughton, 1957), 130.
2. R. Smith, 'Fifty Years of Randomised Controlled Trials', *British Medical Journal*, 317 (1998), 7167.
3. Sir R. Doll, 'Controlled Trials: The 1948 Watershed', *British Medical Journal*, 317 (1998), 1217–20.
4. S.F. Olsen, 'Use of Randomisation in Early Clinical Trials', *British Medical Journal*, 318 (1999), 1352.
5. A.M. Lilienfeld, 'Ceteris Paribus: The Evolution of the Clinical Trial', *Bulletin of the History of Medicine*, 56 (1982), 1–18.
6. The MRC described this study at the time as 'a statistically controlled study... the first of its kind', Medical Research Council, *Report of the*

29

Medical Research Council for the Years 1945–1948 (London: HMSO, 1949), 23.

7. G.B. Hill, 'Controlled Clinical Trials: The Emergence of a Paradigm', *Clinical and Investigative Medicine*, 6 (1983), 25–32.

8. Lilienfeld, *op. cit.* (note 5). Daniel challenged his king to prove that his royal diet was superior to that of his slaves, by comparing the outcome between two groups fed upon the two different diets.

9. J.P. Bull, 'The Historical Development of Clinical Therapeutic Trials', *Journal of Chronic Diseases*, 10 (1959), 218–48; E. Gehan and N.A. Lemak, *Statistics in Medical Research: Developments in Clinical Trials* (New York: Plenum Medical Book Co., 1994); S. Lock, 'The Randomised Controlled Trial: A British Invention', in G. Lawrence (ed.), *Technologies of Modern Medicine* (London: The Science Museum, 1994), 81–7; S.J. Pocock, 'Chapter 2: The Historical Development of Clinical Trials', in S.J. Pocock, *Clinical Trials: A Practical Approach* (Chichester: John Wiley, 1983), 14–27; A.K. Shapiro and E. Shapiro, *The Powerful Placebo: From Ancient Priest to Modern Physician* (Baltimore: Johns Hopkins University Press, 1997), especially Ch. 6, 'The History of Clinical Trials'.

10. Pocock, *ibid.*

11. Bull, *op. cit.* (note 9).

12. Shapiro and Shapiro, *op. cit.* (note 9).

13. See particularly Gehan and Lemak, *op. cit.* (note 9).

14. Fisher's most influential work was probably R. Fisher, *The Design of Experiments* (Edinburgh: Oliver and Boyd, 1935)

15. U. Tröhler, *'To Improve the Evidence of Medicine': The Eighteenth Century British Origins of a Critical Approach* (Edinburgh: Royal College of Physicians of Edinburgh, 2000).

16. M. Meldrum, *'Departures from Design': The Randomized Clinical Trial in Historical Context, 1946–1970* (PhD thesis: State University of New York at Stony Brook, 1994).

17. A. Maehle, *Drugs on Trial: Experimental Pharmacology and Therapeutic Innovation in the Eighteenth Century* (Amsterdam: Rodopi, 1999).

18. J.R. Matthews, *Quantification and the Quest for Medical Certainty* (Princeton: Princeton University Press, 1995). A further discussion of the application of statistics to therapeutic experimentation follows in Chapter 6 of this work.

19. See for example G. Weisz, 'From Clinical Counting to Evidence-Based Medicine', in G. Jorland, A. Opinel and G. Weisz (eds), *Body Counts: Medical Quantification in Historical and Sociological Perspective* (Montreal: McGill-Queen's University Press, 2005), 377–93; also later in this chapter for a related brief discussion of the tensions between clinical and laboratory medicine.

20. Matthews, *op. cit.* (note 18), 145.

21. I. Hacking, 'Telepathy: Origins of Randomization in Experimental Design', *Isis,* 79 (1988), 427–51.

22. T. Dehue, 'Deception, Efficiency, and Random Groups: Psychology and the Gradual Origination of the Random Group Design', *Isis,* 88 (1997), 653–73.

23. Lock, *op. cit.* (note 9).

24. T. Kaptchuk, 'Intentional Ignorance: A History of Blind Assessment and Placebo Controls', *Bulletin of the History of Medicine,* 72 (1998), 389–433.

25. I. Chalmers, 'Comparing Like with Like: Some Historical Milestones in the Evolution of Methods to Create Unbiased Comparison Groups in Therapeutic Experiments', *International Journal of Epidemiology,* 30 (2001), 1156–64; I. Chalmers, 'Statistical Theory was not the Reason that Randomization was used in the British Medical Research Council's Clinical Trial of Streptomycin for Pulmonary Tuberculosis', in G. Jorland, A. Opinel and G. Weisz (eds), *Body Counts: Medical Quantification in Historical and Sociological Perspectives* (Montreal: McGill-Queen's University Press, 2005), 309–34.

26. Alternation means that subjects are allocated to control or treatment groups alternately, in the order in which they present. This is discussed further in Chapter 4.

27. B. Toth, *Clinical Trials in British Medicine 1858–1948, with Special Reference to the Development of the Randomised Controlled Trial* (PhD thesis: University of Bristol, 1998).

28. *Ibid.*

29. A.Y. Yoshioka, *Streptomycin, 1946: British Central Administration of Supplies of a New Drug of American Origin with Special Reference to Clinical Trials in Tuberculosis* (PhD thesis: Imperial College, University of London, 1998).

30. D.C.T Cox-Maksimov, *The Making of the Clinical Trial in Britain, 1910–1945: Expertise, The State and the Public* (PhD thesis: Cambridge University, 1998).

31. H.M. Marks, 'Notes from the Underground: The Social Organization of Therapeutic Research', in R.C. Maulitz and D.E. Long (eds), *Grand Rounds: One Hundred Years of Internal Medicine* (Philadelphia: University of Pennsylvania Press, 1988), 297–336.

32. H.M. Marks, *The Progress of Experiment: Science and Therapeutic Reform in the United States, 1900–1990* (Cambridge: Cambridge University Press, 1997).

33. The phrase is widely adopted by historians, and is discussed in A.M. Brandt and M. Gardner, 'The Golden Age of Medicine?' in R. Cooter and J. Pickstone (eds), *Medicine in the Twentieth Century.* (Amsterdam: Harwood, 2000), 21–37, from which article the claims for the 'golden age' which follow are derived; for the impact of laboratory science see also C. Lawrence,

Medicine in the Making of Modern Britain 1700–1920 (London: Routledge, 1994), 72–6.

34. E.H. Ackerknecht, *Therapeutics from the Primitives to the Twentieth Century* (New York: Hafner Press, 1973).

35. J. Goodman, 'Pharmaceutical Industry', in R. Cooter and J. Pickstone (eds), *Medicine in the Twentieth Century* (Amsterdam: Harwood, 2000), 141–54: 145

36. Brandt and Gardner, *op. cit.* (note 33).

37. G. Risse, 'The History of Therapeutics', in W.F. Bynum and V. Nutton (eds), *Essays in the History of Therapeutics* (Amsterdam: Rodopi, 1991), 3–11.

38. Lawrence, *op. cit.* (note 33), 75.

39. For example, Rosenberg in C.E. Rosenberg, 'The Therapeutic Revolution: Medicine, Meaning, and Social Change in Nineteenth-Century America', in M.J. Vogel and C.E. Rosenberg (eds), *The Therapeutic Revolution: Essays in the Social History of American Medicine* (Pennsylvania: University of Pennsylvania Press, 1979), 3–25, 5, and Warner in J.H. Warner, *The Therapeutic Perspective: Medical Practice, Knowledge and Identity in America, 1820–1885* (Princeton: Princeton University Press, 1997), 4, argue that therapeutic systems prior to the twentieth century – which would nowadays be deemed ineffective – did 'work' within the context of the understanding of health, disease and therapy at the time. Nancy Demand applies the same argument to the efficacy of Hippocratic treatment, N. Demand, 'Did the Greeks Believe in the Efficacy of Hippocratic Treatment – and, if so, Why?' in I. Garofalo, *et al.* (eds), *Aspetti della Terapia nel Corpus Hippocraticum* (Florence: Olschki, 1999).

40. C. Lawrence, 'Clinical Research', in J. Krige and D. Pestre (eds), *Science in the Twentieth Century.* (Amsterdam: Harwood, 1997), 439–59: 444.

41. G. Graham, 'The Formation of the Medical and Surgical Professorial Units in the London Teaching Hospitals', *Annals of Science,* 26 (1970), 1–22.

42. D. Fisher, 'The Rockefeller Foundation and the Development of Scientific Medicine in Great Britain', *Minerva,* XVI (1978), 21–41.

43. Lawrence, *op. cit.* (note 40), 446–7.

44. Marks, *op. cit.* (note 32).

45. See for example, Editorial, 'The Medical Research Council', *British Medical Journal,* i (1925), 225–6; T. Lewis, 'Research in Medicine: Its Position and Needs', *British Medical Journal,* i (1930), 479–83; J.A. Gunn, 'Remarks on the Outlook of Research on Therapeutics', *British Medical Journal,* ii (1932), 389–92.

46. Marks, *op. cit.* (note 32), 31; for examples of studies employing this notion of hospital scrutiny and control over environmental factors such as diet and exercise see for example, W.R. Snodgrass and T. Anderson, 'Prontosil in the Treatment of Erysipelas: A Controlled Series of 312 Cases', *British Medical*

Journal, ii (1937), 101–4; J. F. Wilkinson, 'The Value of Extracts of Suprarenal Cortex in the Treatment of Addison's Disease', *Lancet,* ii (1937), 61–70.

47. See for example, Sir B. Moynihan, 'The Relation of Medicine to the Natural Sciences', *Lancet,* i (1925),115–7, 117; T. Horder, *Health and a Day* (London: J. M. Dent, 1937), 209; J.P. Lockhart-Mummery, 'The Royal Society Discussion on "Experimental Production of Malignant Tumours"', *Lancet,* ii (1933), 323; R. Hutchinson, 'Fashions and Fads in Medicine', *British Medical Journal,* i (1925), 995–8.

48. This account of the MRC, and the details which follow, are derived from A. Landsborough Thomson, *Half a Century of Medical Research. Volume One: Origins and Policy of the Medical Research Council (UK)* (London: HMSO, 1973); A. Landsborough Thomson, *Half a Century of Medical Research. Volume Two: The Programme of the Medical Research Council (UK)* (London: Medical Research Council, 1987); J. Austoker, 'Walter Morley Fletcher and the Origins of a Basic Biomedical Research Policy', in J. Austoker and L. Bryder (eds), *Historical Perspectives on the role of the MRC.* (Oxford: Oxford University Press, 1989), 23–33.

49. Joan Austoker credits him with dominating the development and expansion of medical science in Britain, Austoker, *ibid,* 23; Landsborough Thomson regards him as undoubtedly the principal architect of the MRC, Thomson, *Half a Century of Medical Research Volume 1, ibid,* 228.

50. Fletcher, *op. cit.* (note 1), this is Fletcher's biography by his daughter, Maisie Fletcher.

51. This brief biography is extracted from H.H. Dale, 'Sir Walter Fletcher', *British Medical Journal,* i (1933), 1085–6; Fletcher, *op. cit.* (note 1); Obituary, 'Sir Walter Fletcher', *British Medical Journal,* i (1933), 1085.

52. For Fletcher's own exposition of these views see for example, W. Fletcher, 'Royal Dental Hospital: Address', *British Medical Journal,* ii (1927), 655–6, and W. Fletcher, 'An Address on the Scope and Needs of Medical Research', *British Medical Journal,* ii (1932), 43–7. His opinions, and those of other MRC members, are also described in his biography, *op. cit.* (note 1), particularly 178–9, 194, 246. See also Austoker, *op. cit.* (note 48); J. Liebenau, 'The MRC and the Pharmaceutical Industry: The Model of Insulin', in J. Austoker and L. Bryder (eds), *Historical Perspectives on the role of the MRC.* (Oxford: Oxford University Press, 1989), 163–80; Landsborough Thomson 1987, *op. cit.* (note 48).

53. Austoker, *op. cit.* (note 48), 25.

54. Landsborough Thomson 1973, *op. cit.* (note 48), 40.

55. *Ibid.,* 72.

56. *Ibid.,* 11.

57. Fletcher to Locker Lampson 5/5/1923, Cancer Research Campaign archive

CRC X1/1071; quoted in Austoker, *op. cit.* (note 48), 29.

58. Quoted in J. Austoker, *A history of the Imperial Cancer Research Fund 1902–1986* (Oxford: Oxford University Press, 1988), 86.

59. *Ibid.,* 86; Austoker, *op. cit.* (note 48), 29.

60. Austoker, *op. cit.* (note 48), 30.

61. R. Stevens, *Medical Practice in Modern England* (New Haven: Yale University Press, 1966), 33–7.

62. D. Cantor, 'The MRC's Support for Experimental Radiology during the Inter-War Years', in J. Austoker and L. Bryder (eds), *Historical Perspectives on the Role of the MRC* (Oxford: Oxford University Press, 1989), 181–204.

63. Austoker, *op. cit.* (note 58), 149.

64. *Ibid.,* 149.

65. *Ibid.,* 150.

66. Quoted in *ibid.,* 151.

67. C. Lawrence, 'Incommunicable Knowledge: Science, Technology and the Clinical Art in Britain 1850–1914', *Journal of Contemporary History,* 20 (1985), 503–20.

68. G.L. Geison, 'Divided we Stand: Physiologists and Clinicians in the American Context', in M. Vogel and C. Rosenberg (eds), *The Therapeutic Revolution: Essays in the Social History of American Medicine* (Pennsylvania: University of Pennsylvania Press, 1979), 67–90.

69. S. Sturdy, 'From the Trenches to the Hospitals at Home: Physiologists, Clinicians and Oxygen Therapy, 1914–30', in J. Pickstone (ed.), *Medical Innovations in Historical Perspective* (Basingstoke: Palgrave MacMillan, 1992), 104–23.

70. R.C. Maulitz, '"Physician versus Bacteriologist": The Ideology of Science in Clinical Medicine', in M. Vogel and C. Rosenberg (eds), *The Therapeutic Revolution: Essays in the Social History of American Medicine* (Pennsylvania: University of Pennsylvania Press, 1979), 91–107.

71. J. Parascandola, 'The Search for the Active Oxytocic Principle of Ergot: Laboratory Science and Clinical Medicine in Conflict', in E. Hickel and G. Schröder (eds), *Neue Beiträge zur Arzneimittelgeschichte,* Vol. 51 of *Veröffentlichungen der Internationalen Gesellschaft für Geschichte der Pharmazie e. V.* (Stuttgart: Wissenschaftliche Verlagsgesellschaft, 1982), 205–27.

72. Geison, *op. cit.* (note 68).

73. S. Sturdy and R. Cooter, 'Science, Scientific Management, and the Transformation of Medicine in Britain c. 1870–1950', *History of Science,* 34, 4 (1998), 421–66.

74. Liebenau, *op. cit.* (note 52).

75. Cox-Maksimov, *op. cit.* (note 30), Ch. 3.

76. Cantor, *op. cit.* (note 62).

77. Cox-Maksimov, *op. cit.* (note 30), Ch. 4.

78. Medical Research Council, *Report of the Medical Research Council for the Year 1930–1931* (London: HMSO, 1932), 23.

79. *Ibid.*, 22.

80. Annotations, 'Clinical Trials of New Remedies', *Lancet*, ii (1931), 304; the same announcement was published simultaneously, with almost identical wording, in the *British Medical Journal*.

81. Cox-Maksimov, *op. cit.* (note 30), chapter 5.

82. *Ibid.*, 193.

83. Landsborough Thomson, 1973, *op. cit.* (note 48), 238.

84. Meldrum, *op. cit.* (note 16), 13.

85. This statement arises from my examination of studies published by the TTC and listed in Medical Research Council, *Report of the Medical Research Council for the Year 1932–1933* (London: HMSO, 1934); Medical Research Council, *Report of the Medical Research Council for the Year 1933–1934* (London: HMSO, 1935); Medical Research Council, *Report of the Medical Research Council for the Year 1934–1935* (London: HMSO, 1936); Medical Research Council, *Report of the Medical Research Council for the Year 1935–1936* (London: HMSO, 1937); Medical Research Council, *Report of the Medical Research Council for the Year 1936–1937* (London: HMSO, 1938); Medical Research Council, *Report of the Medical Research Council for the Year 1937–1938* (London: HMSO, 1939); Medical Research Council, *Report of the Medical Research Council for the Year 1938–1939* (London: HMSO, 1940).

86. For example, J.B. Christopherson and M. Broadbent, 'Ephedrine and Pseudo-Ephedrine in Asthma, Bronchial Asthma, and Enuresis', *British Medical Journal*, i (1934), 978–9.

87. For example, Snodgrass and Anderson, *op. cit.* (note 46); T. Anderson, 'Sulphanilamide in the Treatment of Measles', *British Medical Journal*, i (1937), 716–18.

88. Alternation means that patients were allocated alternately to treatment or untreated groups in the order in which they presented to the physician. For example, W.R. Snodgrass and T. Anderson, 'Sulphanilamide in the Treatment of Erysipelas: A Controlled Series of 270 Cases', *British Medical Journal*, ii (1937), 1156–9.

89. For example, Spence in 1933 compared twelve treated subjects with three controls in his investigation of calciferol in the treatment of rickets; he also split two pairs of twins, allocating just one twin in each pair to receive calciferol. J.C. Spence, 'Clinical Tests of the Antirachitic Activity of Calciferol', *Lancet*, ii (1933), 911–15.

90. For example, H.S. Banks, 'Chemotherapy of Meningococcal Meningitis', *Lancet*, ii (1939), 921–6.

91. For example, E.J. Wayne, 'Clinical Observations on Two Pure Glucosides of

Digitalis, Digoxin and Digitalinum Verum', *Clinical Science,* 1 (1933), 63–76.

92. For example, J.F. Wilkinson and M.C.G. Israels, 'The Pentnucleotide Treatment of Agranulocytic Angina', *Lancet,* ii (1934), 353–5.

93. For example, J.S. Maxwell, 'The Treatment of Post-Operative Retention of Urine with "Doryl"', *Lancet,* i (1937), 263–4.

94. For example, L. Colebrook *et al.,* 'Treatment of 106 Cases of Puerperal Fever by Sulphanilamide', *Lancet,* ii (1937), 1237–42 and 1291–3.

95. For example, C. Moir, 'The Use of "Doryl" (Carbaminoyl-choline) in Post-Operative and Post-Partum Retention of Urine', *Lancet,* i (1937), 261–3, the author points out that particularly detailed case reports were kept in order to prepare this report.

96. For example, S.L. Cummins, 'Merthiolate in the Treatment of Tuberculosis', *Lancet,* ii (1937), 962–3.

97. For example, Wilkinson, *op. cit.* (note 46).

98. Toth, *op. cit.* (note 27), 191.

99. *Ibid.,* 170.

100. *Ibid.,* 191.

101. Cox-Maksimov, *op. cit.* (note 30), 192.

102. Toth, *op. cit.* (note 27), 62.

103. Yoshioka, *op. cit.* (note 29).

104. Cox-Maksimov, *op. cit.* (note 30), 71.

105. *Ibid.,* 98.

106. Cantor, *op. cit.* (note 62), 190.

107. Meldrum, *op. cit.* (note 16), 373.

108. J. Schuster and R. Yeo, 'Introduction', in J. Schuster and R. Yeo (eds), *The Politics and Rhetoric of Scientific Method* (Dordecht & Boston: Kluwer, 1986), ix–xxxvii, xx.

109. *Ibid.,* xxvi.

110. R. Yeo, 'Scientific Method and the Rhetoric of Science in Britain, 1830–1917', in J. Schuster and R. Yeo (eds), *The Politics and Rhetoric of Scientific Method* (Dordrecht: Kluwer, 1986), 259–97.

111. M. Pera, 'The Role and Value of Rhetoric in Science', in M. Pera and W. Shea (eds), *Persuading Science: The Art of Scientific Rhetoric* (Canton: Science History Publications, 1991), 29–54.

112. J. Golinski, *Making Natural Knowledge: Constructivism and the History of Science* (Cambridge: Cambridge University Press, 1998).

113. *Ibid.,* 118.

114. P. Kitcher, 'Persuasion', in M. Pera and W. Shea (eds), *Persuading Science: The Art of Scientific Rhetoric* (Canton: Science History Publications, 1991), 3–27.

115. *Ibid.,* 24.

116. C. Bazerman, *Shaping Written Knowledge: The Genre and Activity of the*

Experimental Article in Science (Madison: University of Wisconsin Press, 1988).

117. *Ibid.,* 320.

118. S.L. Montgomery, *The Scientific Voice* (New York: Guilford Press, 1996).

119. *Ibid.,* 45 (his italics).

120. G. Lakoff and M. Johnson, *Metaphors We Live By* (Chicago: University of Chicago Press, 1980).

121. 'Introduction' in R. Williams, *Keywords* (London: Fontana, 1988).

122. R. Young, *Darwin's Metaphor: Nature's Place in Victorian Culture* (Cambridge: Cambridge University Press, 1985).

123. *Ibid.,* 124–5.

124. R. Smith, *Inhibition: History and Meaning in the Sciences of Mind and Brain* (London: Free Association Books, 1992).

125. *Ibid.,* 17.

126. C. Lawrence and R. Dixey, 'Practising on Principle: Joseph Lister and the Germ Theories of Disease', in C. Lawrence (ed.), *Medical Theory, Surgical Practice: Studies in the History of Surgery* (London: Routledge, 1992), 153–215.

127. The following meanings of 'control' are derived from the *Oxford English Dictionary,* 2nd edition (Oxford: Clarendon Press, 1989)

128. Smith, *op. cit.* (note 124), Ch. 2.

129. J. Scott and G. Marshall, 'Scientific Management', in *A Dictionary of Sociology, Oxford Reference Online* (Oxford: Oxford University Press, 2005).

130. S. Bennett, 'The Industrial Instrument: Master of Industry, Servant of Management: Automatic Control in the Process Industries, 1900–1940', *Technology and Culture* 32, 1 (1991), 69–81.

131. E.T. Morman (ed.), *Efficiency, Scientific Management and Hospital Standardization: An Anthology of Sources* (New York: Garland, 1989).

132. S. Timmermans and M. Berg, *The Gold Standard: The Challenge of Evidence-Based Medicine and Standardization in Health Care* (Philadelphia: Temple University Press, 2003), Chapter 1.

133. W. Coleman, *Biology in the Nineteenth Century: Problems of Form, Function, and Transformation.* (Cambridge: Cambridge University Press, 1977), 156.

134. The terms are Boring's, see E.G. Boring, 'The Nature and History of Experimental Control', *American Journal of Psychology,* 67 (1954), 573–89; the account which follows is largely based upon his analysis.

135. See also T. Dehue, 'From Deception Trials to Control Reagents: The Introduction of the Control Group about a Century Ago', *American Psychologist,* 55, 2 (2000), 264–8. Dehue attributes priority to the American psychologist John Coover.

136. Boring makes this point, *op. cit.* (note 134); see also Chalmers, *op. cit.* (note 25).

137. Annotations, *op. cit.* (note 80).

138. Toth, *op. cit.* (note 27), 246.

139. Marks, *op. cit.* (note 32), 31.

140. Cox-Maksimov, *op. cit.* (note 30), 201.

141. For example, M. Kenney *et al.*, 'p-aminobenzenesulphonamide in Treatment of Bacterium Coli Infections of the Urinary Tract', *1 Lancet,* ii (1937), 119–25, described in a *BMJ* Editorial, 'Sulphanilamide in Urinary Infections', *British Medical Journal,* ii (1937), 589–90, as 'the first adequate and controlled study' of sulphanilamide in urinary infections; the study involved extensive laboratory work, but no clinical comparison subjects. See also my later chapter on raw pancreas therapy.

142. For example, Snodgrass and Anderson, *op. cit.* (note 88); Spence, *op. cit.* (note 89); further examples are discussed in my later chapters.

143. *Daily Mail,* 20 November 1943, quoted in Cox-Maksimov, *op. cit.* (note 30), 233.

144. Cox-Maksimov, *op. cit.* (note 30), 204.

2

Good, Bad or Offal?
The Rhetoric of Control in the
Evaluation of Raw Pancreas Therapy

In 1922, Robert Lawrence (1892–1968) was using a small chisel to obtain chippings from a specimen of mastoid bone[1]. A fragment flew into his eye; the ensuing infection was so overwhelming that he was permanently blinded on that side. His colleagues at King's College Hospital soon discovered why this trivial injury had resulted in such a devastating infection. At the age of thirty, the young house surgeon had developed severe diabetes. Aware of the death sentence which this implied at the time, Lawrence retired to Florence in order to spend his remaining months surrounded by the art and culture he adored. However, his artistic contemplation was interrupted by news of the advent of insulin therapy. Returning at once to England he became, in May 1923, one of the first diabetics to receive the new treatment. He was to devote the remainder of his professional life, as a clinician and biochemist, to the investigation and treatment of diabetes.

Lawrence might have had good reason to be an enthusiast for the insulin treatment which had saved his life. He had less truck with raw pancreas therapy, which enjoyed a resurgence in popularity during 1925 as a potential alternative to insulin in the treatment of diabetes. In this year, Lawrence and his allies entered into a debate with the enthusiasts for raw pancreas over the efficacy of the therapy.

Here I explore the raw pancreas debate as an illustration of a wider conflict, between self-styled scientifically-minded doctors and their more clinically-orientated colleagues, over the use of the rhetoric of science in the assessment of a treatment's efficacy. Specifically, the debate centred around the use of the term 'controlled' in describing trials or experiments. The protagonists did not define the word 'controlled', nor do the technical meanings with which they apparently invested it entirely account for the assumptions underlying their use of the term. Rather, the term 'controlled' was largely employed as a rhetorical device to indicate an acceptable trial, conducted by the right kind of scientifically-orientated practitioners who had associations with the MRC.

Figure 2.1

Robert Lawrence (1892–1968).
Courtesy: Wellcome Library, London.

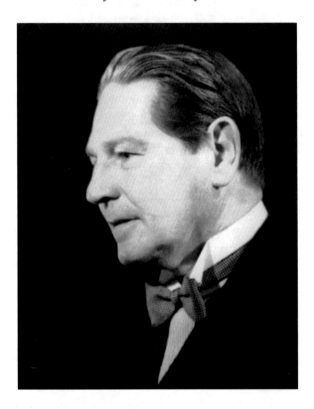

Pancreas therapy and diabetes

The raw pancreas debate occupied the correspondence columns of the *British Medical Journal (BMJ)* from March 1925 to April 1926, and it is these pages which form the core source material for this analysis. No comparable discussion occurred in other contemporary medical journals of record, such as the *Lancet*; possibly the general practitioners (GPs) and provincial consultants who advocated the therapy felt that the readership of the *BMJ* would be more likely to include jobbing physicians who would be sympathetic to their views. I address a British debate, which I situate within the context of British therapeutic reform. There may well be parallels with activity elsewhere, particularly in the United States where the efficacy of raw pancreas and other forms of organ therapy was being scrutinised and where a parallel debate regarding the proper means to demonstrate therapeutic efficacy was conducted. The *Journal of the American Medical Association* (*JAMA*) reflected practitioners' uncertainty, as its editorial position varied from outright condemnation of raw pancreas therapy[2] to acceptance that it could have a role.[3] Contributors to the American debate might well have divided along similar lines to the British protagonists, whom I characterise below as 'scientific' or 'bedside' practitioners. However, in the absence of any significant published historical analysis which provides a global view of early twentieth-century therapeutic reform I have chosen to restrict this study to the UK.

The pancreas was first implicated in the aetiology of diabetes in 1889, when Oskar Minkowski, rather to his surprise,[4] rendered a dog severely diabetic by removing its pancreas. The administration of pancreatic tissue to diabetic patients might, some physicians reasoned, replace the missing pancreatic ingredient and control the disease. Over the next few years practitioners reported cases in which they administered pancreatic juice or extracts, by mouth or injection, to their diabetic patients, or fed them raw or cooked pancreas. The first to claim success was the Massachusetts physician William Cowles, who performed his experiment in 1897 although he neglected to publish it for a further fourteen years. He ascribed his therapeutic success to his patient's ability to consume an unprecedented quantity of pancreas – up to six raw calves' pancreases every day, cut into pieces the size of an oyster and bolted whole. Cowles claimed that the diabetes did not reappear until his patient ate a stale specimen which provoked vomiting and left him disgusted, whereupon he refused to swallow any more pancreas, with fatal consequences.[5]

Most investigators' results were generally negative or inconclusive, however, and pancreatic organotherapy was largely abandoned by the early-twentieth century. Even the hypothesis that the pancreas was implicated at all in the aetiology of diabetes, remained controversial,[6] until the discovery of insulin placed the pancreas squarely back in the frame. The isolation of insulin from the pancreas in 1921 and its successful application to the treatment of diabetes from 1922, established a rational basis for pancreatic organotherapy and provoked another flurry of enthusiasm for the treatment.[7] Oral pancreatic therapy offered potential advantages over insulin, which was expensive – one physician considered in 1924 that 'At present only the millionaire or insurance patient can afford insulin.'[8] Sufficient raw pancreas for four days' treatment could, however, be had for eight pence[9] – the equivalent cost for insulin would have been around six to twelve shillings.[10] Enthusiasts also suggested that oral therapy was safer, as there was no risk of the potentially fatal hypoglycaemia which could afflict patients on insulin[11] and more convenient, as unlike insulin therapy it did not necessitate two or more injections every day.[12] Tattersall[13] describes how the need for multiple daily injections was initially regarded as a major obstacle to insulin therapy, particularly as few physicians believed that patients could be entrusted with their own injections.

Mackenzie Wallis, a chemical pathologist at St Bartholomew's Hospital, claimed in 1922 to have perfected a technique for preparing a stable, orally effective pancreatic extract administered in gelatin capsules.[14] First and foremost a laboratory scientist who had obtained his medical degree in 1913 only after several years of part-time study, he was fascinated by pancreatic pathology and was the first to devise a means of estimating blood glucose from a fingerprick blood sample.[15] His extract was subsequently produced commercially by the drug firm Parke Davis. However, it was three years later, with a description from a GP of the results of raw pancreas therapy, that the debate over oral treatment resurfaced.

The clamour for raw pancreas, 1925

Thomas Hollins was an Irish-born Chesterfield GP, with a fondness for golf.[16] He re-ignited the controversy over the role of raw pancreas with an article in the *BMJ* in March, 1925. In the course of the ensuing debate, doctors were to cajole scores of diabetic patients into consuming the unappetising preparation. Indeed patients themselves, learning of the rediscovered therapy, started 'clamouring for raw pancreas'[17] – although Lawrence, who had developed firm views on the unpalatability of the disgusting raw preparation after trying it upon himself, commented that the only patients so clamouring were those who had not yet tried it.[18]

Hollins[19] recounted his experience with seven patients whom he claimed to have successfully treated with pancreas and gave detailed case reports for two. He concluded that a tablespoon of the raw minced gland every day was sufficient to lower blood sugar to acceptable levels – though he mentioned only one actual blood sugar estimation – and to abolish the excretion of glucose and ketones in the urine. Taken with lettuce, the minced preparation formed a 'delicious meal' which diabetic patients appeared naturally to crave. Free from the 'grave risks', such as hypoglycaemia, and irksome injections attendant on insulin therapy, he considered that the raw gland represented an effective, and frequently superior, substitute for insulin.

Support for Hollins's experience followed, predominantly from GPs. Two weeks after Hollins's account, Dr Robertson Young described his experiments with raw pancreas thirty years previously. Inspired by 'The success which in those early days attended the administration of thyroid gland in myxoedema,' he had administered raw pancreas to 'some half-dozen' diabetics, with favourable effects on their symptoms, weight, wellbeing and urinary glucose excretion. He had prepared the gland in exactly the same fashion as Hollins, finely minced and mixed with lettuce, and successfully presented his results to gain his MD.[20] Shortly afterwards, William Dunn, a Rutland physician and school medical officer,[21] described a 21-year-old diabetic man whom he had successfully treated with raw pancreas. Given the prohibitive cost of insulin, he considered that the use of pancreas 'is of even greater practical importance than that of insulin, as it brings the treatment within the range of the mass of people.'[22]

The first to publish dissent was Geoffrey Harrison, a biochemist colleague of Lawrence's who had worked on diabetes at King's College and Great Ormond Street Hospitals, supported by a grant from the MRC.[23] Unimpressed by the observations of the previous correspondents, he chose to repeat their experiments 'under carefully controlled conditions'. He described two patients, providing a table of blood sugar estimations for one, and details of the rigid diet to which they were subject. Raw pancreas, he concluded, had no effect – any apparent benefit had probably been due to alterations in the patients' diets once they started pancreas therapy.[24]

George Graham, a physician at St Bartholomew's Hospital, reinforced Harrison's negative findings. The author of a number of articles on the pathology of diabetes, he too undertook work on diabetes under the auspices of the MRC, and had been one of the workers involved in the 1923 MRC study of the therapeutic use of insulin.[25] He described the results of raw pancreas therapy on a 14-year-old girl, providing details of her diet and tables of daily blood sugar. He concluded that the therapy was useless.[26]

GPs continued to argue in favour of pancreas therapy. Two female practitioners, Helena Pomeroy Kelly from Wolverhampton[27] and Constance Griffiths from Cardiff,[28] each described a single patient in whom they had used it with success. Then, in May 1925, Hollins, the originator of the controversy, responded to the negative findings of Harrison and Graham. Raw pancreas, he claimed, was only effective in patients who had never received insulin, though he admitted that he was at a loss to explain why this should be so. Harrison and Graham's patients had previously received insulin therapy, which explained the lack of effect when they were treated with pancreas. Hollins rejected Harrison's suggestion that the apparent benefit of pancreas was due to concomitant dietary modification and insisted that his patients had been 'most carefully dieted for some months.'[29]

At this point Lawrence entered the fray. Choosing to investigate the effect of pancreas therapy upon himself, he discontinued his own insulin and forced down an ounce of raw gland before lunch, before dinner, at bedtime, and again the next morning. The therapy was disgusting – even 'a dozen injections a day' would have been preferable – and failed to regulate his diabetic symptoms or his blood sugar. He promised a further, 'carefully controlled' experiment to verify this negative finding.[30] This 'controlled' experiment followed one month later, supported by Lawrence's grant from the MRC. Lawrence described two patients who consumed one ounce of raw pancreas every day – they disliked the gland intensely, despite its being disguised in a sandwich. He presented detailed descriptions of his patients' diets and tables of urine sugar estimations, to support his conclusion that raw pancreas was completely ineffective.[31]

There followed a case report from Dr Carrasco-Formiguera, a Barcelona paediatrician, who provided detailed tables of dietary intake and urinary sugar excretion to demonstrate that pancreas therapy had been ineffective in a two-and-a-half-year-old diabetic boy. He agreed with Lawrence that 'All duly controlled experiments' had failed to demonstrate any advantage of pancreas therapy.[32] Despite its profusion of detail – and its being one of only three contributions to the debate to appear as a *BMJ* article rather than as correspondence[33] – this Spanish report was not referred to again throughout the controversy.

Jack Bernstein, a Preston GP, then offered to 'help clear up the matter' and presented blood sugar charts from two patients he had treated with raw pancreas.[34] Blood sugar estimations were expensive and not always easy for a GP to obtain – Bernstein acknowledged the help that the pathologist at the local Preston Royal Infirmary had provided in performing these tests for him. The charts, which he deemed 'self-explanatory', documented a decline in blood sugar following the commencement of pancreas therapy and subsequent rise following its cessation, on a number of occasions over a period of several months. Bernstein found his patients quite happy to consume raw pancreas, minced and mixed with green vegetables such as cress or lettuce, and concluded that it was an effective treatment for diabetes. Lawrence's riposte suggested that Bernstein's tables lacked essential details, such as the timing of blood sugar tests in relation to meals, and the nature, duration, and rigidity of his patients' diets. 'In the recent discussion in your columns,' he concluded, '*all* investigators who have carefully controlled *all* the factors have found raw pancreas quite useless.'[35] Bernstein replied immediately, giving details of the timing of blood tests – all were performed three hours after breakfast – and diet, which was 'not rigid' but prohibited sugar, potatoes, and carbohydrate-rich foods.[36]

Percy Cammidge, a physician and bacteriologist with an interest in diabetes, suggested a compromise. In an earlier letter[37] he had proposed that insulin contained not one, but two components, only one of which was effective by mouth. Patients with different types of diabetes manifested different responses to the two components, he claimed, which explained why oral therapy appeared to work in some patients and not in others. In a further article[38] he described experiments with rats which, he claimed, supported his theory. He referred to his own 'clinical experience' with

Figure 2.2
Advertisement for a polyglandular preparation, 1925

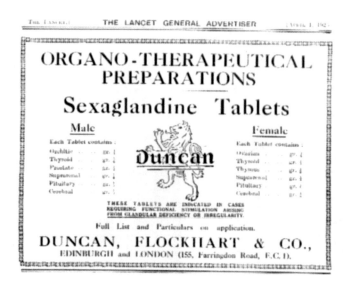

various pancreas preparations, particularly Mackenzie Wallis extract, which supported his assertion that oral pancreas therapy *was* effective, but only in the right type of diabetic.

A case report from Ernest Neve, senior surgeon at the Kashmir Mission Hospital, provided the final item of support for raw gland therapy. A 16-year-old boy with newly diagnosed diabetes failed to respond to insulin; his doctors decided to try raw pancreas instead. Initially there was no improvement, until Neve realised that 'what was being given was not pancreas' – precisely which internal organ was being administered, the surgeon does not record. Once the proper gland was substituted, the boy made a rapid recovery.[39] Cunningham Affleck, an Edinburgh physician, shared Neve's frustration with the idiosyncrasies of butchers and slaughterhouse workers. He discovered that they generally supplied thymus or thyroid glands in place of pancreas when asked for 'sweetbreads'. It was necessary, he cautioned, to specify 'long bread' or 'gut bread' in order to receive pancreas. Those who had found pancreas unpleasant had probably been supplied with the wrong organ, for true pancreas was 'quite pleasant and palatable'. Indeed, he suggested that it was sometimes difficult to acquire, as the slaughterhouseman frequently purloined it from the carcass as a delicacy for himself.[40]

There the correspondence ended, ultimate victory apparently falling to the opponents of pancreas therapy. Raw pancreas does not appear to have been advocated any further in print, advertisements for pancreatic preparations disappeared from medical journals,[41] and commercial production of Mackenzie Wallace's pancreatic extract had ended by 1928.[42] By 1931, the *Lancet* could look back upon what its editorialist described as:

> [A] long and it must be confessed dismal history of various pancreatic preparations which when given by mouth were claimed to effect a reduction in the blood-sugar and urine-sugar content... a distressing chapter in the story of endocrinology.[43]

Organotherapy in 1920s Britain

Treatment with organ extracts – organotherapy – was widespread, though not uncontroversial, in Britain at the time of this debate. George Murray's successful use, in 1891, of thyroid extract to treat hypothyroidism had encouraged physicians over the subsequent three decades to experiment with a variety of other extracts. Besides pancreatic organotherapy in the treatment of diabetes, physicians administered preparations derived from ductless and digestive glands, testicles, ovaries, prostate, breast, nerve, muscle, and other tissues in the treatment of a large number of conditions. Critics pointed out that disorders selected for organotherapy were frequently rather vaguely defined,[44] and extracts from testicles and ovaries appeared to feature particularly prominently amongst the ingredients of many commercially available preparations.

Organotherapy rapidly became associated, by some physicians, with quackery and reckless empiricism. Prominent amongst the critics were laboratory-orientated practitioners, particularly those investigating the biochemistry and physiology of hormones in the newly emergent speciality of endocrinology, such as Edward Sharpey-Schäfer, Swale Vincent, and Ernest Starling. They claimed that empirical glandular therapy was ineffective, as it lacked any rational scientific basis; indeed, to Vincent it represented a threat to the whole field of endocrinology.[45] Sharpey-Schäfer warned of 'the defects of mere clinical observation, unassisted by experimentation on animals'[46] in assessing its therapeutic value, and Vincent considered most organotherapy 'a formidable kind of quackery'.[47] Alfred Clark, Professor of Therapeutics at University College London, singled out for particular ridicule the practice of administering a cocktail of extracts from a number of different organs. Such polyglandular therapy was, he considered, 'as far removed from rational therapy as is the writing out of a charm on a piece of paper and giving that to the patient to swallow.'[48] These

Figure 2.3
Advertisement for a polyglandular preparation, 1925

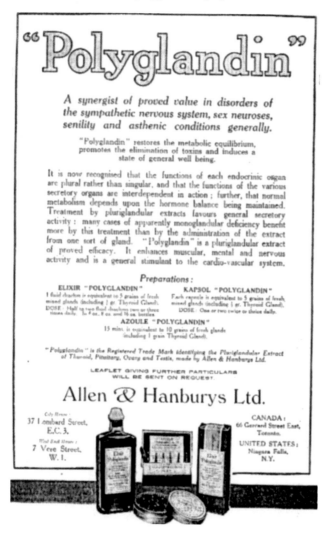

critical laboratory scientists frequently considered that the GP bore much of the blame for over-enthusiastic administration of organ extracts. One physician, while praising the restraint of 'Scientific investigators with critical minds,' selected for opprobrium 'a mass of general practitioners, most dispensing chemists, a number of consultants, not a few journalists, many oriental medical men'[49] who chose to adopt such remedies. Nevertheless, many GPs and some, mainly provincial, consultants continued to prescribe organotherapy on the basis that it was popular and appeared to work in practice, irrespective of experimental or laboratory findings.[50]

Reflecting in 1937 on the state of endocrine therapy during the first quarter of the century, the editor of the *BMJ* noted that various gland extracts had then been 'prescribed with an enthusiasm that outran knowledge. Indiscriminate endocrine therapy brought about the inevitable reaction, and clinical endocrinology came to be looked upon with suspicion.'[51] Nevertheless, the new science of endocrinology flourished; Merriley Borell describes how the study of internal secretions came to prominence 'in spite of the over-zealous prescription of organ extracts by practitioners and the subsequent development of an uneasy alliance between physicians and laboratory scientists.'[52]

Drug firms saw organotherapy as an opportunity for potential profit, and promoted it accordingly. Unsurprisingly, scientifically-minded practitioners railed against them, too – Clark considered that through the efforts of 'commercial enterprise... endocrine therapy is coming to bear a suspicious resemblance to mediaeval magic....'[53] An anonymous physician castigated: 'Certain of the firms placing "endocrine" preparations on the market', who 'have realised the commercial possibilities in exploiting the human weakness' of the gullible,[54] and Vincent lamented that 'certain... manufacturing druggists are... growing rich by reason of the inadequate education of medical practitioners and the notorious ignorance of the general public....'[55] Nevertheless, the *Lancet* and *BMJ* carried weekly advertisements for such preparations, from isolated extracts of testicles, ovaries, and other organs, to polyglandular preparations available off-the-shelf or manufactured to individual physicians' specifications.

Scientists and clinicians in the pancreas debate

The protagonists in the conflict over raw pancreas divide along similar lines to those involved in the broader organotherapy debate. Those who opposed raw pancreas therapy may be characterised as MRC-sponsored, laboratory-orientated, academically-minded 'physician–biochemists'. Its supporters were jobbing bedside clinicians. This division between clinicians and scientists has been the subject of recent scholarship and is particularly reminiscent of Christopher Lawrence's analysis of the increasing application of laboratory science to clinical medicine during the early-twentieth century. He argues that enthusiasts for laboratory techniques were countered by 'patrician' clinicians who valued individual bedside clinical acumen which, they said, could only arise from broad learning, proper upbringing, and extensive clinical experience.[56] These practitioners ascribed a more minor role to laboratory tests in the context of their clinical work. The 'scientific' practitioners sought to render laboratory work very much to the fore.

The opponents of raw pancreas therapy may be characterised as the laboratory orientated, scientific physicians of Lawrence's analysis. Notably, they all had affiliations to the MRC, which made no secret of its commitment to fundamental laboratory science in clinical research. Robert Lawrence, Harrison, and Graham were firmly in the MRC camp. All were recipients of MRC grants to support their work on diabetes and Lawrence was a member of the MRC research staff. He and Harrison were trained as biochemists, had been colleagues in the biochemistry department of King's College Hospital, and worked jointly on diabetic research for the MRC.[57] Both maintained a laboratory-orientated, scientific concept of their clinical work. Lawrence, at this time, was concerned mainly with laboratory research work into diabetes rather than practical patient care[58] and Graham, 'one of the early physician biochemists... a laboratory physician,' was committed to 'teaching scientific medicine to students and applying physiological principles at the bedside.'[59] As the following analysis will demonstrate, these biochemist–physicians did not validate their opinions regarding therapeutic efficacy through clinical experience alone. Rather, their claims were based upon what they perceived as the proper use of laboratory science and employed a distinct style of presentation and rhetoric.

The supporters of raw pancreas therapy were, on the other hand, an assortment of jobbing bedside clinicians. Most were GPs, though Neve was a surgeon in Kashmir and Dunn held a post at Rutland County Hospital, besides acting as medical officer for a couple of schools and for the local post office. Cammidge had previously held a post as a county bacteriologist in the West Riding.[60] These bedside practitioners validated their opinions regarding therapeutic efficacy through their own clinical experience and observations. The GP Hollins referred to 'many theoretical objections' to pancreas therapy, and enumerated three – that digestion would destroy the gland's active principle; that previous experiments had failed to demonstrate any clinical benefit; and that it was difficult to ensure that the correct part of the gland was being administered. He dismissed these arguments simply by appealing to his own observations: 'In spite of these and other objections the use of raw fresh gland has yielded such striking results during the two and a half years I have been using it that I think they are worth recording.'[61] To Helena Pomeroy Kelly, clinical experience ranked over rationale or research: 'From experience I think it too unsafe to be dogmatic on any line or treatment for diabetes, as, despite recent research, the aetiology and pathology of some cases are most puzzling and they refuse to respond to any form of treatment.'[62] Cammidge, despite presenting some animal experiments, was ultimately convinced of the effectiveness of raw pancreas therapy by 'My clinical experience with various preparations of pancreas.'[63] Neve considered that the effect of raw pancreas in his case report was 'decisive' and that the numerous positive case reports published lent strong support to its use, despite the objections of Lawrence's camp.[64]

The advocates of raw pancreas also relied upon their clinical experience for the correct way to administer the therapy. Hollins even blamed the physician–biochemists' lack of therapeutic success upon their failure to observe strictures born of experience. He stressed that the gland must be perfectly fresh: 'In this I think lies the explanation of the failure of other observers to obtain any useful results with raw gland,'[65] and that it must be raw.[66] His justification for these claims was entirely empirical. Cunningham Affleck cautioned, through his experience, how difficult it could be to obtain true pancreas and gave instructions on how to specify the correct organ in butcher's parlance.[67] The biochemist–physicians preferred to counter the GPs' empiricist arguments with scientific rationale. Whereas Hollins cheerfully admitted that he was 'at a loss to explain'[68] his observation that raw pancreas was ineffective in diabetics who had previously received insulin, Lawrence responded with a detailed explanation based upon the physiological effects of sudden cessation of insulin therapy.[69]

Central to what the protagonists were actually arguing *about*, was the properly controlled status of the experiments produced as evidence. Consistently, the biochemist–physicians criticised the 'uncontrolled' nature of their opponents' submissions and contrasted their own 'well controlled' studies. On no occasion did any of the protagonists attempt to define what they meant by 'controlled', although the term certainly did not refer to its present-day meaning of an untreated comparison group – none of the reports in this controversy featured one, or made any reference to its desirability. Nor was the appropriateness of a 'controlled' experiment in question – the GP Hollins, in response to Harrison's criticism, declared himself 'anxious that this treatment may be subjected to the most rigid and carefully controlled tests.'[70] However, the biochemist–physicians' use of the term ultimately aimed to reserve it exclusively for their own work.

The meaning of 'controlled': control and the patient's environment

Among the implicit technical meanings with which the protagonists in this debate invested the term 'controlled', were a careful regulation of patients' diets and other environmental factors, and the validation of investigators' claims by laboratory data. The biochemist Harrison decided to repeat Hollins's and Young's inadequately controlled experiments 'under carefully controlled conditions'.[71] Although he did not define 'controlled', his report differed from that of the previous authors in its quantification of the nutritional components of his patients' diets – grams per day of carbohydrate, protein, and fat – and the provision of a table of blood sugar estimations for one patient. Graham, too, when he supported Harrison's conclusions, provided similar nutritional details and tables of blood sugar readings for his patient. Lawrence also considered 'controlled' experiments to be crucial and used the term at least partly to encompass dietary control, 'in carefully controlled cases on *weighed* and constant *quantitative* diets, raw pancreas is no substitute for insulin.'[72] He promised a 'carefully controlled experiment' to test the matter; this appeared as a description of two diabetic women, with details of their nutritional intake and a chart of urinary glucose excretion.[73] His concept of 'controlled' clearly included other factors besides dietary control – he found it necessary to stress that '*all* investigators who have carefully controlled *all* the factors have found raw pancreas quite useless'[74] and that it was essential that 'the diet *and other factors* are fully controlled'[75] in any such experiment.

The *BMJ* also called for 'controlled' experiments in organotherapy. An editorial marking the publication of a new book, *Glandular Therapy*, bemoaned the tendency of physicians to try glandular therapies which 'lack any support from controlled experiments...'.[76] *Glandular Therapy's* section on oral pancreas therapy considered that a 'controlled' experiment principally involved laboratory measurements – pancreas therapy was dismissed as ineffective after being submitted 'to the scrutiny of clinical tests controlled with simultaneous laboratory investigation.'[77]

This notion of control as regulation of environmental factors such as diet, and validation by laboratory tests, would appear to concord with Marks's and Cox's analyses of the term.[78] However, the analysis which follows demonstrates that these criteria alone are insufficient to define the 'controlled' experiment in the raw pancreas controversy. Comparing the biochemists' 'controlled' experiments with the 'uncontrolled' investigations of the raw pancreas enthusiasts reveals that the methodology of both groups of practitioners was broadly similar – both administered pancreas to small numbers of selected diabetic patients and documented the results. The remainder of this chapter will demonstrate that the differences between the two sets of accounts largely related to the means by which results were presented and claims were validated, and to the criteria adopted to define therapeutic success.

Diet – do you believe me?

The bedside clinicians responded to the biochemists' criticisms that their experiments were inadequately controlled. Harrison had suggested that Hollins's patients improved because of an alteration in their diet rather than due to pancreas therapy. Hollins rejected this notion, declaring that his patients had previously 'been most carefully dieted for some months both by me personally and at the local hospital.'[79] Constance Griffiths similarly pointed out that 'no change was made in the diet' of her patient,[80] Helena Pomeroy Kelly maintained that her patient had been subject to a 'strict diet',[81] and Ernest Neve claimed that his patient was subject to the strict Allen starvation diet.[82]

One of the criteria which the biochemist–clinicians expected of a properly controlled trial of therapy in diabetes, was strict adherence to an unchanging, prescribed diet. Harrison kept his patients' diet 'fixed rigidly',[83] Graham's was 'constant'[84] and Lawrence's was 'fixed'.[85] It was not, however, sufficient simply to claim that this criterion had been fulfilled – the statement, according to the biochemist–clinicians, had to be backed up by quantitative details. Hollins, Griffiths, Pomeroy Kelly, and Neve simply stated that their patients' diets had remained unchanged. Even when challenged, Hollins apparently considered that a reply stating that his patient had been dieted 'most carefully... by me personally'[86] would be sufficient, without providing quantitative detail. Nevertheless, the GPs' bald statement – unsupported by quantitative data – that the diet was unchanged, was insufficient to persuade the biochemists that their trials were properly controlled. Lawrence required detail, 'we are told that a "strict diet" was observed, but are given no details and are not even assured that it was weighed.'[87] Without such detail, there was no defence against the suggestion that any therapeutic effect was due to a change in diet: 'the supporters, by giving no facts or figures, lay themselves open to this accusation.'[88]

These biochemists and bedside practitioners were making the same claim – that their patients' diets had remained unchanged throughout the experiment. Their rhetoric, however, was different. The bedside clinicians expected their word, supported by their status and clinical experience, to stand. The biochemists expected their statements to be validated by detail – grams per day of carbohydrate, protein, and fat intake – as exemplified by their descriptions of their own experiments. Steven Shapin has described the emergence, during the seventeenth century, of criteria to establish the trustworthiness of a witness to an experimental phenomenon. Gentlemen, of appropriate background and education, and obeying careful rules of presentation and discourse, were regarded as particularly credible witnesses. To disbelieve their testimony would be discourteous – today, it remains impolite to discredit expert experience: 'It is at least uncivil, and perhaps terminally so, to decline to take knowledge from authoritative sources.'[89] The GPs in the pancreas debate relied simply upon their status as physicians to give credence to their experimental claims, in accordance with established practice and rules of presentation.[90] Nevertheless, the biochemist-physicians performed the discourtesy of discounting the GPs' claims. The rhetorical device they employed to justify their incivility, was to label the GPs' work inadequately controlled.

The meaning of disease control

Not all the bedside clinicians aimed to maintain their patients on a constant diet. Indeed, some argued that the fact that patients' strict diets could be relaxed once they started raw pancreas, was evidence for the therapy's success. Bernstein made this claim, stating, 'both patients were allowed substantial amounts of ordinary white bread after being on raw pancreas a short time, with no apparent ill results.'[91] Young, too, found that it was no longer 'necessary to enforce too strict a diabetic diet'[92] once his patients had started pancreas therapy, and Dunn's patient, thanks to raw pancreas, was able to consume a 'full ordinary diet (bread, potatoes, milk puddings) and there is not a trace of sugar in the urine.'[93] These statements illustrate a difference in approach to another meaning of the term 'control', in relation to the *clinical* control of disease. Diabetes could not be cured; instead, both groups of practitioners aimed for disease 'control'. However, such disease control was interpreted differently by the two groups. To the bedside practitioners, it implied primarily the alleviation of *symptoms*, with biochemical data merely providing a degree of support. To the biochemist–clinicians, disease control implied the achievement of normal, or acceptable, results of laboratory biochemical tests.

The GPs detailed their patients' improving symptoms as evidence of the therapy's success. Hollins described his patients' subjective wellbeing and the effect of diabetes upon the job of one, the foreman in an ironworks.[94] Young described the therapy's effect upon symptoms of thirst, polyuria and general wellbeing;[95] Pomeroy Kelly's patient became 'wonderfully better, her abnormal thirst and appetite having practically disappeared,'[96] Griffiths found that therapy caused 'all symptoms to disappear',[97] and Neve's patient was symptomatically 'much improved'.[98] The biochemist–physicians, Harrison, Graham, Lawrence, and Carrasco-Formiguera gave no details whatsoever concerning their patients' symptoms, instead referring exclusively to biochemical analysis of blood or urine.[99] This 'biochemical' concept of control necessarily implied strict control of diet, without which it would be impossible to interpret changing blood and urinary sugar levels. To the bedside clinicians, disease control was synonymous, to a far greater extent, with *symptom* control. Dietary laxity was therefore permissible, providing it did not compromise the patient's subjective wellbeing.

The notion that scientifically-minded practitioners redefined their concepts of disease according to laboratory criteria, is not new. Tattersall[100] has analysed physicians' attitudes to diabetes control following the advent of insulin therapy. He describes the 'chemical school'[101] who strove to maintain their patients' blood sugar constantly as near-normal as possible, through strict diet and close monitoring of insulin dosage, and those physicians who allowed dietary laxity in favour of a superior quality of life. Chris Feudtner has highlighted the same debate in the United States following the isolation of insulin and uses detailed case reports powerfully to illustrate the moral associations of diabetes control, whereby both the physicians who prescribed severely restrictive diets and the patients who complied with them were considered to be exercising virtuous traits.[102] Olga Amsterdamska[103] discusses the development, early in the twentieth century, of biochemical techniques to monitor and re-describe in physiological terms, activities such as the workings of the kidney. These techniques ultimately contributed towards a redefinition of some diseases according to biochemical rather than clinical criteria. Keith Wailoo has described a similar effect of novel technologies and emergent specialities in helping to redefine both diseases and the nature of effective treatments, in haematological conditions such as chlorosis and splenic anaemia.[104]

These different notions of disease control might reflect, in part, the different relationships with their patients enjoyed by the bedside practitioners and biochemist–clinicians. GPs had to pay for laboratory access, and most rarely used such investigations. They did, however, face potential competition for patients, both state-funded 'panel' patients and the more lucrative private clientele.[105] Keeping their customers happy and loyal made good business sense, and GPs might well have preferred to judge a preparation's therapeutic efficacy by its ability to relieve symptoms or improve subjective wellbeing, thereby ensuring a satisfied customer, in preference to biochemical parameters, and when patients wanted such treatment, there was financial incentive for the GPs to comply – unlike the salaried biochemist Lawrence, who felt equipped to resist his patients' 'clamouring for raw pancreas'.[106] The biochemist–physicians might have considered that such pecuniary interest in the success of a compound could compromise the GPs' objectivity when it came to assessing its efficacy.[107] Raw pancreas was also an inexpensive remedy, within the financial grasp of many panel patients for whom insulin would have been prohibitively expensive.

The biochemist–physicians, on the other hand, might have had a number of reasons to eschew accounts of their patients' symptoms in their assessment of therapeutic efficacy. Their salaried status provided some separation from the financial incentives which influenced the GPs. Although many would also have undertaken private work, they clearly separated their experimental work on hospital patients, from private practice – Harrison, for example, specifically distinguished his different use of diet and insulin 'In *experimental* work' from that 'In *ordinary practice*'.[108] The GPs' emphasis on symptoms and case histories might also have reminded the biochemists of the widespread use, by drug companies in their promotional material, of personal testimonials from satisfied patients and practitioners. These testimonials were the source of suspicion amongst scientifically-minded practitioners.

At the time of the pancreas controversy, convenient blood sugar estimation – even on fingerprick blood samples – was becoming available, at least in hospital practice,[109] and urine analysis for glucose was routine.[110] The biochemist–physicians in this debate appear to have redefined clinical control in diabetes according to such biochemical criteria. By these biochemical standards, the bedside clinicians were incapable of demonstrating that they had achieved proper disease control; their trials therefore could not be properly controlled in the eyes of the biochemist–physicians. These scientific practitioners would not accept dietary laxity, or therapeutic outcome measures based primarily upon symptomatic improvement. These, according to their own notions of disease control, signified an inadequately controlled trial. Both groups could conceivably have claimed that theirs was the proper use of the term 'control' in relation to disease suppression; in practice, it was the biochemists who adopted the term as their own.

Laboratory control and how to present it

The bedside clinicians did, nevertheless, provide some biochemical data to support their claims that raw pancreas therapy was effective. All described the effect of therapy upon urine sugar levels, apart from Bernstein who described exclusively blood sugar estimations. In addition, Hollins undertook one blood sugar reading. Their urine sugar results were not presented in tables, but incorporated into the textual description of their patients' case histories – either as a simple statement that the urine 'contained sugar' or was 'sugar free',[111] or as a quantitative estimation of the percentage of sugar in the urine.[112] By contrast, the biochemists all presented their results in tabular form. Harrison and Graham presented tables of blood sugar estimations, Lawrence and Carrasco-Formiguera tabulated urine glucose readings.[113] The biochemical investigators' aspiration for 'clinical tests controlled with simultaneous laboratory investigation' has already been mentioned; meticulous tabulation was part of the proper presentation of such careful laboratory control, as opposed to the narrative descriptive style of the bedside clinicians. Amsterdamska similarly mentions the importance to American biochemists, of presenting their findings exclusively as tables and graphs without further textual comment.[114]

Bernstein,[115] however, differs from the other GPs in that he appears to have presented his findings in a fashion very similar to the biochemists. Unlike his pro-pancreas colleagues, he gave no account of his patients' symptoms. He presented the results for his two patients as graphs of blood sugar levels measured while they were taking, and not taking, raw pancreas. He refrained from comment upon the charts 'which I believe are self-explanatory...' and which ostensibly demonstrated a fall in blood sugar when the patients were taking raw pancreas and a rise when they abandoned it.

However, Bernstein's account still did not satisfy the biochemists' expectations for laboratory or dietary control. Lawrence criticised Bernstein for failing to describe his patients' diets, or the time – in relation to meals – that the blood tests were performed. Bernstein's study was therefore uncontrolled. Lawrence went on to conclude that '*all* investigators who have carefully controlled *all* the factors have found raw pancreas quite useless.'[116] Bernstein replied[117] with details of diet and the timing of blood sugar tests, which were all taken three hours after breakfast; Lawrence remained unimpressed.[118]

Even when Bernstein presented his data in a fashion analogous to the biochemists, his study was deemed inadequately controlled. Bernstein's graphical presentation of his results was ostensibly meticulous and apparently conveyed equivalent information to the biochemists' own tables. His use of blood sugar estimations as the sole measure of disease activity conformed with the biochemists' notions of biochemical rather than clinical disease control – and blood sugar estimations were widely accepted as a more rigorous control measure than the urine analysis which was employed by Lawrence.[119] His avoidance of any description of his patients' symptoms, and his invitation to readers to draw their own conclusions from his results, accorded with the biochemists' presentational style. Only in the criteria he used to defend the charge that his patients' diets could have varied did he fail to conform to the biochemists' expectations. His study was nevertheless deemed inadequately controlled. Bernstein was a GP; he stood little chance of his study being accepted as 'controlled' by the scientifically minded practitioners who sought to adopt the term as their own.

Self experiment or controlled experiment?

One episode which fits a little oddly into this analysis, is Lawrence's initial description of his experience when he tried raw pancreas therapy himself.[120] On 27 May 1925, he stopped his insulin; maintaining a constant diet, he forced down four ounces of 'horrible' raw pancreas over the next twenty-four hours. He recorded fifteen separate blood sugar levels during this time, and specified his daily diet – 45 grams of carbohydrate, 80 grams of protein, 150 grams of fat. He did not, however, present this self-experiment as 'controlled' despite its apparently accommodating the factors which characterised the biochemists' controlled experiments – it was performed by a biochemist, with meticulous descriptions of diet and of biochemical data. Lawrence himself implied that it was not controlled when he promised to follow it up with 'a carefully controlled experiment' and when he concluded that raw pancreas was ineffective, not because of the self-experiment he had just described, but on the basis of previously published 'carefully controlled cases....'[121] Nor was this self-experiment referred to again throughout the controversy, by Lawrence or anyone else.

Lawrence also presented his self-experiment in a different fashion to the biochemists' other controlled trials. He provided the only description of symptoms in any of the biochemists' accounts – his own 'thirst and polyuria were severe' on the morning after he started the experiment – and his numerous blood and urine sugar estimations were incorporated into the textual narrative of his own case history rather than being accommodated into a table. He was not, it seems, adopting the rhetoric which he considered appropriate to the presentation of a properly controlled trial, and apparently did not consider his self-experiment to be such. It was more in the way of a personal account.

He also elaborated at length upon just how disgusting he found the therapy to be. Previous authors had already attested to its unappetising nature; Cowles, in his description of the first successful attempt at therapy, attributed his success to his patient's ability to swallow an unprecedented quantity of the unappealing gland, until an experience with a stale pancreas resolved him to consume no more.[122] Lawrence found the experience of consuming pancreas 'so horrible as to prefer a dozen injections a day.' He attributed any success it might have, to an improvement in diet, due to the disinclination of a patient who has consumed raw pancreas to eat any other food!'[123] In his subsequent 'controlled' experiment, he disguised the pancreas in a sandwich, but nevertheless his patients 'disliked [it] very much.'[124] Otherwise the biochemists made no reference to the palatability of the therapy.

The enthusiasts did, however, refer to the acceptability of raw pancreas, and painted a very different picture. Hollins's patients found that pancreas made a 'delicious meal'[125] when taken with lettuce, Young administered it 'without... any disinclination to take it on the part of the patient',[126] and Bernstein's patients 'assure me that they have become quite accustomed to the mixture.'[127] These claims were not substantiated or debated, but were simply presented as representations of the subjective impressions of the patients receiving the therapy. Once again, the bedside clinicians expected their word to stand. Lawrence felt able to dispute their claims on the basis of his own subjective experience. Conceivably, Lawrence might have felt less inclined to credit the bedside clinicians' evidence when these experiences concorded so poorly with his own. Nevertheless, in describing his disgust at pancreas therapy he was adopting the style more appropriate to a bedside clinician's narrative case history than to a biochemist's controlled trial.

This self-experiment, then, was not 'controlled'. This is unlikely to be due to any lack of methodological rigour; indeed, the degree of control which the meticulous Lawrence could exert over his own diet, therapy, and biochemical testing could be considerably greater than that which he could exert over his patients.[128] It is not the lack of such dietary and environmental regulation which deprived this self-experiment of its 'controlled' status.

Self-experimentation enjoyed a rather mixed reputation at the time. On the one hand was the heroic, self-sacrificial, solitary, romantic image of the medical self-experimenter. Schaffer describes the association of self-experiment with the emergent notion of the romantic, scientific genius at the beginning of the nineteenth century.[129] In an editorial, the *BMJ* in 1926 still portrayed figures such as Rivers, who damaged his ulnar nerve in order to investigate its re-growth, and Haldane and Barcroft who inhaled dangerous concentrations of gases, as heroic loners in the pursuit of truth.[130] Ebstein, writing in 1931, concluded: 'at all times numerous physicians were ready to sacrifice their lives for the promotion of science and the benefit of their fellow-men... they deserve to be remembered as shining examples.'[131] Walter Reed and his team performed self-experiments on yellow fever early in the twentieth century and were portrayed not only in scientific articles but also in contemporary plays, films, novels, and paintings as selfless, courageous heroes.[132] On the other hand, a more disreputable image simultaneously attached to self-experimentation. Danger to the experimenter – and lack of objectivity – were commonly cited. Altman mentions contemporary criticism of self-experimenters such as Daniel Carrion[133] who was accused of bringing disgrace upon the medical profession when he fatally inoculated himself, towards the end of the nineteenth century, with Oroya fever in order to prove its link with skin lesions known as verrugas; and Werner Forssmann,[134] who performed the first cardiac catheterisation procedure upon himself in 1922. He was reprimanded by his superior and subsequently failed to gain a post as a result of the reputation which attached to him following his self-experiment. Late-nineteenth-century self-experiments with mind-altering preparations including nitrous oxide, ether, cocaine, and cannabis had also created a number of addictions and left the reputation of self-experimentation tarnished.[135]

Lawrence might, then, have had reason to feel uncomfortable with his self-experiment. The narrative style in which he presented it, with details of symptoms and without tabulated data, might suggest that he regarded this as a subjective account, lacking the objectivity of a third-person study. But in inquiring why it did not entirely fulfil his expectations for a properly controlled trial, it might also be instructive to examine another significant therapeutic development in the treatment of diabetes – the isolation and production of insulin. The biochemist–physicians considered that insulin represented a triumph for their methodology and for the application of basic scientific principles to medicine. Specifically, the model they applauded for the development and exploitation of insulin, involved teamwork and co-ordinated efforts by many researchers. Lawrence wrote of 'a series of brilliant researches by many investigators culminating in the recent discovery of insulin. It is a story of which mankind and scientific effort may well be proud.'[136] Professor J.J.R. Macleod attributed the isolation of insulin to 'excellent team work'[137] and a *BMJ* editorial described the 'co-ordinated team in close touch with the National Institute for Medical Research at Hampstead'[138] who would be responsible for the investigation into the uses of insulin in Britain. The *Lancet* emphasised that information gained by these researches would be shared amongst all participating researchers,[139] and the *BMJ* described how Macleod's observations had 'been extended over a wide range by a team of collaborators.'[140]

Altman, in his analysis of the history of medical self-experimentation, suggests that the rise of the drug companies early in the twentieth century led to therapeutic research being conducted increasingly by teams, resulting in less scope for the lone self-experimenter: 'No longer spirited amateurs making discoveries in private pharmacies and laboratories, they became professional, paid to work as members of large teams.'[141] Lawrence[142] and Marks[143] similarly point to the rise of teamwork during early-twentieth century therapeutic innovation. If teamwork – exemplified by the insulin story – was the biochemist–physicians' model for therapeutic progress, then the solitary, heroic figure of the lone self-experimenter might not accommodate easily to it. The diffidence with which Lawrence began his account could suggest that he was not entirely comfortable with his role as hero: 'May I, as a diabetic, enter the arena in the important discussion that has been going on in your columns...?'[144] His self-experiment did not fit the collaborative model he admired and could not rank alongside properly controlled investigations.

Conclusion

The scientific practitioners involved in the raw pancreas debate systematically employed the term 'controlled' at least partly as a rhetorical device to validate their own accounts. The protagonists in the debate represented two disparate groups. One valued clinical experience and personal testimony, the other, the rhetoric and means of presentation appropriate to laboratory science. Frequently, the two groups were making equivalent claims regarding, for example, the biochemical validation of their results, and their aim for a constant diet. But the groups differed in their use of clinical experience and patients' symptoms – versus laboratory analysis – to validate disease control; the proper way to verify therapeutic claims, such as a constant diet; and the proper way to present biochemical findings. The biochemist–physicians, by using the term 'controlled' to describe *their* means of fulfilling these criteria, adopted it as their own rhetorical device. It thus became impossible for the bedside clinicians properly to fulfil the criteria, simply because they were not biochemists.

At no point in this debate did the biochemists attempt to define their notion of a 'controlled' trial, though they consistently used the term against their opponents. They had rendered the proper conduct of a therapeutic trial tacit – it could only be adopted by biochemists, who were privy to this tacit knowledge. The consistent criticism by the biochemists that their opponents' work was inadequately controlled, ultimately amounted to a criticism that the work had not been performed by biochemists. The MRC's scientific practitioners had adopted the term, and the powerful rhetorical overtones it conveyed, as a weapon in the competition to establish themselves as the proper arbiters of therapeutic efficacy.

Notes

1. The biographical details which follow are derived from Lawrence's obituary, Obituary, 'Robert Lawrence', *British Medical Journal*, 3 (1968), 621–2, and R.B. Tattersall, 'A Force of Magical Activity: The Introduction of Insulin Treatment in Britain 1922–1926', *Diabetic Medicine* 12 (1995), 730–55.
2. Editorial, 'The Administration of Insulin', *Journal of the American Medical Association*, 81 (1923), 753.
3. Editorial, 'Can Insulin Replace the Pancreas?' *Journal of the American Medical Association*, 84, 15 (April 1925), 1122.
4. M. Nothman, 'The History of the Discovery of Pancreatic Diabetes', *Bulletin of the History of Medicine*, XXVIII (1954), 272–4. Nothman was Minkowski's assistant.
5. W.N. Cowles, 'A Case of Diabetes Treated by Feeding of Calves' Pancreas', *Boston Medical and Surgical Journal*, 74 (1911), 921–2.
6. The history of changing concepts of the role of the pancreas and of oral pancreas therapy is documented by Robert Tattersall, R.B. Tattersall, 'Pancreatic Organotherapy for Diabetes 1889–1921', *Medical History* 39 (1995), 288–316; see also H.H. Dale, 'A Lecture on the Physiology of Insulin', *Lancet*, i (1923), 989–93; J.J.R. Macleod, 'Insulin and Diabetes', *British Medical Journal*, ii (1922), 833–5.
7. C.B.S Fuller, 'Oral administration of Pancreatic and Other Preparations in Diabetes', *British Medical Journal*, i (1928), 798–800, 798.
8. J.A. Nixon, 'Diabetes and Insulin', *British Medical Journal*, i (1924), 53–5.

9. W. Dunn, 'Treatment of Diabetes by Raw Fresh Gland (Pancreas)', *British Medical Journal*, i (1925), 680.

10. Assuming a daily consumption of 25–50 units and a price of 6s. 8d for 100 units in 1924. Editorial, 'The Price of Insulin', *British Medical Journal*, i (1924), 339.

11. This advantage of oral therapy was cited by a number of contemporary authors including Hollins, T.J. Hollins, 'Treatment of Diabetes by Raw Fresh Gland (Pancreas)', *British Medical Journal*, i (1925), 503–4, and Dunn, *op. cit.* (note 9).

12. Hollins, *ibid.*, described insulin injections as 'troublesome and irksome'.

13. Tattersall, *op. cit.* (note 1).

14. R.L. Mackenzie Wallis, 'The Internal Secretion of the Pancreas and its Application to the Treatment of Diabetes Mellitus', *Lancet*, ii (1922), 1158–61.

15. Obituary, 'R. L. Mackenzie Wallis', *British Medical Journal*, i (1929), 710–11.

16. *Medical Who's Who*. (7th edn, London: The London & Counties Press Association Ltd, 1925).

17. R.D. Lawrence, 'Raw Pancreas by Mouth Compared with Insulin', *British Medical Journal*, i (1925), 1108.

18. *Ibid.*

19. Hollins, *op. cit.* (note 11).

20. R. Robertson Young, 'Treatment of Diabetes by Raw Fresh Gland (Pancreas)', *British Medical Journal*, i (1925), 632.

21. *Medical Directory* (London: John Churchill and Sons, 1925).

22. Dunn, *op. cit.* (note 9).

23. For example, he acknowledged both the MRC grant and his close co-operation with Lawrence, in G.A. Harrison, 'Can Insulin Produce even a Partial Cure in Human Diabetes Mellitus?', *Quarterly Journal of Medicine*, 1925, 223–34.

24. G.A. Harrison, 'Treatment of Diabetes by Raw Fresh Gland (Pancreas)', *British Medical Journal*, i (1925), 760–1.

25. G. Graham and C.F. Harris, 'The Treatment of Diabetes Mellitus with Insulin and Carbohydrate Restriction', *Lancet*, i (1923), 1150–3. Here, Graham details case reports which also constituted part of the MRC report, Medical Research Council, 'Report to the Medical Research Council: Insulin and the Treatment of Diabetes: Some Clinical Results', *Lancet*, i (1923), 905–8.

26. G. Graham, 'Treatment of Diabetes by Raw Fresh Gland (Pancreas)', *British Medical Journal*, i (1925), 859–60.

27. H. Pomeroy Kelly, 'Treatment of Diabetes by Raw Fresh Gland (Pancreas)', *British Medical Journal*, i (1925), 921.

28. C. Griffiths, 'Treatment of Diabetes by Raw Fresh Gland (Pancreas)', *British Medical Journal*, i (1925), 921.
29. T.J. Hollins, 'Treatment of Diabetes by Raw Fresh Gland (Pancreas)', *British Medical Journal*, i (1925), 946–7.
30. Lawrence, *op. cit.* (note 17).
31. R.D. Lawrence, 'Raw Pancreas by the Mouth in the Treatment of Diabetes', *British Medical Journal*, ii (1925), 87.
32. R. Carrasco-Formiguera, 'Treatment of Diabetes by Raw Fresh Gland (Pancreas)', *British Medical Journal*, ii (1925), 552–3.
33. The others were Hollins's original article, Hollins, *op. cit.* (note 11), and Cammidge's animal experiments, P.J. Cammidge, 'The Effects of Pancreas Preparations by the Mouth upon Carbohydrate Metabolism', *British Medical Journal*, ii (1925), 1216–18.
34. J. Bernstein, 'Raw Pancreas by Mouth Compared with Insulin', *British Medical Journal*, ii (1925), 844.
35. R.D. Lawrence, 'Raw Pancreas by Mouth Compared with Insulin', *British Medical Journal*, ii (1925), 920, his italics.
36. J. Bernstein, 'Raw Pancreas by Mouth Compared with Insulin', *British Medical Journal*, ii (1925), 979.
37. P.J. Cammidge, 'Treatment of Diabetes by Raw Fresh Gland (Pancreas)', *British Medical Journal*, i (1925), 805.
38. Cammidge, *op. cit.* (note 33).
39. E.F. Neve, 'Raw Pancreas in Diabetes Mellitus', *British Medical Journal*, i (1926), 476.
40. C.R. Affleck, 'Raw Pancreas by the Mouth in the Treatment of Diabetes', *British Medical Journal*, i (1926), 727.
41. Tattersall, *op. cit.* (note 6), 312, points to the rapid disappearance of advertisements for such preparations after 1922, following the isolation of insulin.
42. Fuller, *op. cit.* (note 7), confirms that by 1928 the capsules 'have not recently been manufactured.'
43. Editorial, 'Oral Anti-Diabetic Remedies', *Lancet*, i (1931), 31–2.
44. S. Vincent, 'The Present Position of Organotherapy', *Lancet*, i (1923), 130–2.
45. D. Long Hall, 'The Critic and the Advocate: Contrasting British Views on the State of Endocrinology in the early 1920s', *Journal of the History of Biology*, 9, 2 (1976), 269–85.
46. Obituary, 'E. Sharpey-Schafer', *The Fight Against Disease*, XXIII, 2 (1935), 22–5.
47. Vincent, *op.cit.* (note 44), 131.
48. A.J. Clark, 'The Experimental Basis of Endocrine Therapy', *British Medical Journal*, ii (1923), 51–3, 53.

49. A. Physician, 'Some Thoughts about Endocrinology', *Lancet,* i (1923), 207.
50. See for example, F. Theobalds, 'Polyglandular Therapy', *British Medical Journal,* ii (1923), 209; W. Langdon Brown, 'Endocrine Therapy', *Lancet,* i (1925), 739; S. Vincent, 'The Uses and Abuses of Endocrine Therapy', *Lancet,* ii (1925), 331–2.
51. Editors of the British Medical Journal, *The Endocrines in Theory and Practice: Articles Republished from the British Medical Journal.* (London : H.K. Lewis, 1937). Quote from preface, v.
52. M. Borell, 'Setting the Standards for a New Science: Edward Schafer and Endocrinology', *Medical History,* 22 (1978), 282–90, 284.
53. Clark, *op. cit.* (note 48), 51.
54. A. Physician, *op. cit.* (note 49).
55. Vincent, *op. cit.* (note 44), 131.
56. C. Lawrence, 'Incommunicable Knowledge: Science, Technology and the Clinical Art in Britain 1850–1914', *Journal of Contemporary History,* 20 (1985), 503–20; see the first chapter of this volume for a discussion of the tensions between clinicians and scientists during the early-twentieth century.
57. The MRC first awarded Lawrence a grant of £200 for research into diabetes in 1924, following Harrison's support of Lawrence's application. This grant was renewed annually for over 10 years and increased to finance an assistant. MRC folder FD1/1547 (Public Records Office, London)
58. Obituary, *op. cit.* (note 1).
59. Obituary, 'George Graham', *British Medical Journal,* 4 (1971), 563.
60. Medical Directory, *op. cit.* (note 21).
61. Hollins, *op. cit.* (note 11).
62. Pomeroy Kelly, *op. cit.* (note 27).
63. Cammidge, *op. cit.* (note 37).
64. Neve, *op. cit.* (note 39).
65. Hollins, *op. cit.* (note 11), 503.
66. *Ibid.,* 503.
67. Affleck, *op. cit.* (note 40).
68. Hollins, *op. cit.* (note 29).
69. Lawrence, *op. cit.* (note 17).
70. Hollins, *op. cit.* (note 29), 947.
71. Harrison, *op. cit.* (note 24).
72. Lawrence, *op. cit.* (note 17), his italics.
73. Lawrence, *op. cit.* (note 31).
74. Lawrence, *op. cit.* (note 35), his italics.
75. H. Maclean and R.D. Lawrence, 'Oral Administration of Pancreatic Preparations in the Treatment of Diabetes', *British Medical Journal,* ii (1926), 323–4, quote 323, my italics.
76. Editorial, 'Glandular Therapy', *British Medical Journal,* i (1925), 1137.

77. American Medical Association, *Glandular Therapy* (Chicago: American Medical Association, 1925), 10
78. See chapter 1 of this work
79. Hollins, *op. cit.* (note 29).
80. Griffiths, *op. cit.* (note 28).
81. Pomeroy Kelly, *op. cit.* (note 27).
82. Neve, *op. cit.* (note 39).
83. Harrison, *op. cit.* (note 24), 760.
84. Graham, *op. cit.* (note 26), 859.
85. Lawrence, *op. cit.* (note 31).
86. Hollins, *op. cit.* (note 29).
87. Lawrence, *op. cit.* (note 17).
88. *Ibid.*
89. S. Shapin, *A Social History of Truth: Civility and Science in Seventeenth-Century England.* (Chicago: University of Chicago Press, 1994), 20.
90. As discussed in the first chapter of this volume, case reports from individual physicians remained the primary means of communicating novel therapeutic experience; although debate over the interpretation of findings was permissible, commentators were not expected simply to gainsay the experience of others.
91. Bernstein, *op. cit.* (note 36).
92. Robertson Young, *op. cit.* (note 20).
93. Dunn, *op. cit.* (note 9).
94. Hollins, *op. cit.* (note 11).
95. Robertson Young, *op. cit.* (note 20).
96. Pomeroy Kelly, *op. cit.* (note 27).
97. Griffiths, *op. cit.* (note 28).
98. Neve, *op. cit.* (note 39).
99. The one exception to this statement occurs in Lawrence's description of his self-experiment, where he mentions his own thirst and polyuria. The implications of this are discussed below. Lawrence, *op. cit.* (note 17).
100. R.B. Tattersall, 'The Quest for Normoglycaemia: A Historical Perspective', *Diabetic Medicine* 11 (1994), 618–35.
101. 'Chemical School' was Edward Tolstoi's description of the advocates of strict normoglycaemia; *ibid.,* 625.
102. C. Feudtner, *Bittersweet: Diabetes, Insulin and the Transformation of Illness* (Chapel Hill: University of North Carolina Press, 2003), particularly Chapter 5, 'The Want of Control: Ideas and Ideals in the Management of Diabetes', 121–45.
103. O. Amsterdamska, 'Chemistry in the Clinic: The Research Career of Donald Dexter van Slyke', in S. de Chadarevian and H. Kamminga (eds.), *Molecularizing Biology: New Practices and Alliances, 1910s–1970s*

(Amsterdam: OPA, 1998).

104. K. Wailoo, *Drawing Blood: Technology and Disease Identity in Twentieth Century America* (Baltimore: Johns Hopkins University Press, 1997).
105. A. Digby and N. Bosanquet, 'Doctors and Patients in an Era of National Health Insurance and Private Practice, 1913–1938', *Economic History Review*, 2nd ser., XLI , 1 (1988), 74–94: 91 for remarks on GPs' use of laboratories.
106. Lawrence, *op. cit.* (note 17).
107. Vincent, *op. cit.* (note 44), 130, criticised such optimistic empiricism.
108. Harrison, *op. cit.* (note 24), 761, his italics.
109. By 1924, physicians could reliably estimate glucose from a 0.2ml blood sample taken from a fingerprick, though the technique remained expensive; G.A. Allan, 'Diabetes Mellitus and its Treatment by Insulin', *British Medical Journal*, i (1924), 50–3.
110. *Ibid.*; also Tattersall, *op. cit.* (note 100), 620.
111. Hollins, *op. cit.* (note 11); Young, *op. cit.* (note 20); Dunn, *op. cit.* (note 9).
112. Pomeroy Kelly, *op. cit.* (note 27); Griffiths, *op. cit.* (note 28); Neve, *op. cit.* (note 39).
113. Again, the exception to this general statement is Lawrence's self-experiment, discussed below.
114. See Amsterdamska, *op. cit.* (note 103), 67–8, regarding Donald Van Slyke's presentation of nephritis as a series of graphs representing chemical parameters; also p. 63, with regard to the biochemist Henderson who worked at Harvard and Yale Universities and developed nomograms to represent changes in blood physiology; Henderson feared that 'we should reject one of the most precious advantages of mathematics... if we were to translate into English that which can be well said only in the nomographic idiom.'
115. Bernstein, *op. cit.* (note 34).
116. Lawrence, *op. cit.* (note 35), his italics.
117. Bernstein, *op. cit.* (note 36).
118. He did not refer specifically to Bernstein again, but maintained his opinion that all adequately controlled experiments had discounted the value of pancreas therapy. See Maclean and Lawrence, *op. cit.* (note 75).
119. The advent of insulin therapy led to disagreement amongst practitioners as to whether expensive and inconvenient blood sugar estimations were strictly necessary to assess disease control, but they were nevertheless regarded as superior to urinary estimations. Tattersall, *op. cit.* (note 1), 752; Allan, *op. cit.* (note 109); A. Innes, 'Insulin Treatment Without Blood Sugar Estimations', *British Medical Journal*, i (1924), 55–6.
120. Lawrence, *op. cit.* (note 17).
121. *Ibid.*

122. Cowles, *op. cit.* (note 5), 921.

123. Lawrence, *op. cit.* (note 17).

124. Lawrence, *op. cit.* (note 31).

125. Hollins, *op. cit.* (note 11).

126. Robertson Young, *op. cit.* (note 20).

127. Bernstein, *op. cit.* (note 34).

128. Altman cites this as one advantage of self experimentation, since the highly motivated experimenter is more likely rigidly to control factors such as diet. L.K. Altman, *Who Goes First? The Story of Self-Experimentation in Medicine.* (Berkeley: University of California Press, 1998), 304.

129. S. Schaffer, 'Self Evidence', *Critical Inquiry,* 18 (1992), 327–62.

130. Editorial, 'Auto-Experimenters', *British Medical Journal,* i (1926), 914.

131. E. Ebstein, 'Medical Men who Experimented upon Themselves', *Medical Life,* 38 (1931), 216–18.

132. Described in Altman, *op. cit.* (note 128), 130.

133. *Ibid.,* 4.

134. *Ibid.,* 45–6.

135. *Ibid.,* 57–8, 211–12.

136. R.D. Lawrence, *The Diabetic Life: Its Control by Diet and Insulin* (London: J. & A. Churchill, 1925), 10.

137. Macleod, *op. cit.* (note 6), 833.

138. Editorial, 'The Treatment of Diabetes by Insulin', *British Medical Journal,* ii (1922), 991–2.

139. Editorial. 'The Treatment of Diabetes by Insulin', *Lancet,* i (1923), 391–2.

140. Editorial, 'Insulin and Diabetes', *British Medical Journal,* ii (1922), 882.

141. Altman, *op. cit.* (note 128), 98.

142. C. Lawrence, 'Clinical Research', in J. Krige and D. Pestre (eds), *Science in the Twentieth Century* (Amsterdam: Harwood, 1997), 439–59, see 446–7.

143. H.M. Marks, *The Progress of Experiment: Science and Therapeutic Reform in the United States, 1900–1990* (Cambridge: Cambridge University Press, 1997).

144. Lawrence, *op. cit.* (note 17).

3

Bright Lights, Smoky Cities:
Light Therapy in 1920s Britain

Look here said Sir Walter, by Gad
Ray therapy is utterly bad
We'll set it at naught
In an annual report
This will serve as a Vitaglass ad![1]

In November 1928, King George V spent a pleasant week shooting on his
Sandringham estate. Towards the end of his stay, on Saturday the 17th, he
began to feel feverish and unwell. Nevertheless, he continued to undertake
his duties, attending church the next day and returning to London on the
Monday to hold Council. By Tuesday his condition had deteriorated
sufficiently for him to call his doctors; Sir Stanley Hewett attended him and
promptly sought the opinion of Lord Dawson. The King had developed
pleurisy. His condition rapidly deteriorated and was to cause grave concern
for weeks to come.[2]

Anxiety concerning the monarch's health, and indeed over his very
survival, rapidly spread throughout the British Empire.[3] The King became
too unwell to attend to his duties, and on 4 December a commission of six
counsellors of state was appointed to undertake these on his behalf.[4] An
operation, on Wednesday 12 December, to drain pus from his chest cavity,
left him feeble and exhausted.[5] The following Sunday, his physicians decided
to enlist help from two specialists in a popular, and apparently potent, new
remedy – light therapy.[6]

The King received regular exposure to ultra-violet rays from a mercury
lamp as part of his treatment over the following weeks. Any response to the
therapy appears to have been less than dramatic – he recovered slowly, only
gaining sufficient strength to travel to Bognor for his convalescence in
February 1929[7] and choosing St George's Day to release a message of
gratitude to the nation for his continuing recovery.[8] He was subsequently to
suffer further chest infections, from which he eventually died in 1936.

This episode nevertheless serves to underline the contemporary
prominence of light therapy in mainstream medical practice. Widely
practised, and almost universally acclaimed as therapeutically effective, light

67

therapy in Britain faced its first serious challenge in 1929, when the MRC published two clinical trials which deemed it ineffective. These findings aroused incredulity and opposition from the medical profession. This chapter examines the strategies employed by practitioners in attempting to discredit or discount the conclusion that light therapy lacked proven efficacy, and the means by which the MRC defended its findings, largely by exploiting the rhetoric of a 'controlled trial'. This rhetorical strategy was similar to that described in the previous chapter examining the raw pancreas debate. The audience for the MRC's claims regarding light therapy was, however, different. Whereas the raw pancreas debate represented a spat between physicians, conducted in the pages of a professional medical journal, the light therapy debate was a broader, more public affair. It took place not only in medical journals, in the MRC's own reports, and in meetings of doctors' professional bodies, but also received a considerable amount of coverage in newspapers, whose lay correspondents felt able to comment upon, and to criticise, the conduct of the trials. In addition, the MRC was very much on the attack in the pancreas debate, where it probably represented the mainstream medical opinion against a rather rag-tag collection of practising physicians, who enjoyed little status amongst the prevailing medical elite. Its criticisms of light therapy, by contrast, placed it firmly on the defensive; its findings flew in the face of established mainstream medical opinion, and opposition was swift and vitriolic, often arising from highly regarded physicians. The MRC was caught on the back foot, and employed the rhetoric of control in its defence.

Light therapy in 1920s Britain

The notion that sunlight conveys therapeutic or healing properties enjoys an ancient pedigree and remains pervasive even now.[9] Hippocrates prescribed sunbaths for the treatment of wasted muscles and the Romans made extensive therapeutic use of solaria. The treatment appears to have fallen into some disuse during the early-Middle Ages, possibly due to its association with pagan cults of sun-worship, but resurfaced towards the end of the eighteenth century and became increasingly widespread up to the early-twentieth century.[10] It was during the 1920s, however, that artificial light therapy boomed in Britain.

The increasing popularity of sunlight therapy throughout the nineteenth century was associated with discoveries which suggested a scientific rationale for its therapeutic effects. The presence of an invisible component of sunlight, above the violet end of the spectrum and hence christened ultraviolet radiation, was established in 1801. The ability of light, and in particular this ultraviolet light, to kill bacteria was described in 1877 and this discovery inspired the Danish physician Niels Finsen, in 1894, to experiment for the first time with artificially-produced ultraviolet light in the treatment of the hitherto incurable cutaneous *lupus vulgaris*.[11] His results appeared favourable and his method was adopted with enthusiasm. The therapy reached England in 1901 when Finsen gave a lamp to his Danish compatriot, the Princess of Wales, shortly to become Queen Alexandra, who donated it to the London Hospital; patients came from all over the world to receive the new treatment, sometimes sacrificing their life savings or working their passage.[12]

Artificially generated ultraviolet light therapy enjoyed a steady growth in popularity over the next few years; it was adopted by a number of hospitals in Britain and its reputation spread in the treatment of an increasing number of predominantly dermatological conditions. The new therapy was rarely applied to diseases other than those of the skin, however, possibly being rather sidelined by the apparently more dramatic X-ray therapy,[13] until the start of the 1920s. Then, light therapy boomed and was extended to treat an enormous range of conditions unrelated to diseases of the skin. Artificial light treatment centres appeared in hospitals and other sites across the country, frequently funded by the Ministry of Health or municipal authorities in response to public demand.[14] This surge in popularity appears partly to have been inspired by the demonstration in the early 1920s of real physiological and biochemical effects of ultraviolet light, in particular its effects on calcium and phosphorus metabolism in the skin[15] and subsequently in the skin's manufacture of the newly-discovered vitamin D.[16] In 1922, the MRC established its Committee on the Biological Actions of Light which, largely under the guidance of Leonard Hill and Albert Eidinow at the National Institute for Medical Research, undertook a series of predominantly laboratory-based animal and *in-vitro* experiments. Besides confirming the bactericidal power of ultraviolet light,[17] they demonstrated beneficial effects of ultraviolet irradiation upon leucocyte counts and the bactericidal power of the blood, effects upon proteins in the skin and blood, and upon blood vessels in the skin.[18]

These discoveries provided a scientific rationale for the apparent success of ultraviolet therapy in the treatment of rickets – established by this time as being due to deficiency of vitamin D – and skin infections, but were also interpreted as pointing to the possibility of other, far more wide-reaching benefits. Workers reasoned that since ultraviolet light had been shown to affect some physiological and biochemical processes, it could well exert other, hitherto unknown or inexplicable effects on the body, mediated through its effects on the skin, with the prospect of further therapeutic benefits on a variety of bodily systems.[19] Light therapy expanded rapidly – one commentator dated the 'boom' specifically to around 1925[20] – and became widespread and mainstream. Textbooks could soon list dozens of disparate medical conditions which could benefit including lumbago, rheumatism, gout, 'nervous fidgety states', manic depression, delusional states, Parkinson's disease, asthma, diabetes, high blood pressure, and obesity, besides over thirty separate skin conditions.[21] Even enthusiasts were frequently sceptical about the huge variety of conditions for which light therapists claimed benefit – one noted in 1927 that 'if a list of the diseases said to have benefited was made it would probably begin with acne and go through to zona, including housemaid's knee and minor psychoses'[22] – but they nevertheless remained convinced of the therapy's virtues, concerned only that representing it as a panacea could blind others to its genuine benefits.[23]

The new treatment attracted various synonyms – light therapy, ray therapy, ultraviolet therapy, actinotherapy, and artificial sunlight. Numerous lamps of differing types were commercially available to practitioners and were heavily advertised in the pages of medical journals such as the *British Medical Journal* (*BMJ*) and *Lancet*. Ultraviolet therapy was the most popular, although some physicians chose to combine ultraviolet light with bright white light or infra-red in the treatment of various conditions; others preferred to exclude all visible light, believing that it might actually impair the metabolic effects of ultraviolet.[24] Few voices were raised in opposition to the therapy, although some considered that its psychological component might be more important than was generally realised.[25] Certainly, the treatment must have been impressive; patients were required to strip to their underwear, wear protective goggles, and were exposed either individually or in small groups, to powerful lights which, in the case of arc devices, also emitted noise, smoke, and fumes. Ultraviolet therapy was considered particularly suited to the inhabitants of Britain, suffering as they were from a lack of natural sunlight and 'the smoke cloud which hovers over large cities,'[26] and which robbed city-dwellers of their rightful allocation of ultra-violet rays.[27] Northern cities such as Glasgow were considered particularly deficient in natural sunlight and were regarded as obvious sites for light therapy clinics.[28] Workers whose occupations deprived them of natural light, such as coal miners and even cinema usherettes, were deemed particularly suitable cases for light treatment.

Light therapy also captured the popular imagination during the 1920s. One commentator recalled that at this time 'the public began to demand the treatment for every ill under the sun,'[29] and ultraviolet lamps became widely available for domestic use. Such was the popularity of the new therapy that in May 1928 *The Times* enclosed an entire supplement devoted to the subject.[30] Practitioners without medical qualifications were easily able to acquire ray therapy equipment and set up light clinics, and many did so. Medical practitioners appear generally to have deplored both the domestic use of ultraviolet lamps and even more so their unregulated use by non-medical practitioners. Doctors made frequent calls for light therapy to be controlled, and its use restricted to qualified physicians; such calls emanated not only from light therapists,[31] but were echoed by mainstream medical opinion as exemplified by editorial comment in the *BMJ*.[32] Although physicians generally regarded light therapy as benign, they emphasised its dangers in the hands of unqualified operators and 'the many tyros in the field,'[33] reporting cases where patients treated by such unqualified personnel had suffered harmful effects including eye and skin damage,[34] and even miscarriage.[35] The tragic death of John Jeffrey, a 21-year-old law student who electrocuted himself with an ultraviolet ray lamp he had purchased to treat blackheads on his neck and which he unadvisedly used whilst having a bath,[36] led to further calls for regulation in the medical press.[37] Light therapy frequently came up for discussion during meetings of the British Medical Association, but debate centred largely around the need for its regulation by the medical profession rather than any investigation of its therapeutic merits.[38]

The MRC and light therapy

The rapid expansion in popularity of light therapy appears rather to have caught the MRC by surprise. It had established its Committee on the Biological Actions of Light (CBAL) in 1922, but this was initially concerned with laboratory studies on the biochemical and physiological effects of light rather than validation of any therapeutic effect. In 1925, Dame Janet Campbell and Salisbury MacNalty visited clinics and interviewed practitioners in order to provide a report to the MRC on the current state of clinical light therapy. They concluded that there was evidence of benefit in a number of conditions including cutaneous tuberculosis and a number of other skin conditions, tuberculous peritonitis, tuberculous arthritis, asthma, bronchitis, breastfeeding difficulties, 'dull and backward children', raised blood pressure, leukaemia, and noted the 'tonic effect in over-worked and run-down persons, particularly in adolescents'. However, they pointed out that this evidence was largely anecdotal and emphasised the urgent need for research and control in view of the growing popular demand for the treatment: 'Unfortunately artificial light therapy is having a popular vogue at the present moment and we strongly deprecate the uncontrolled use of lamps for their general therapeutic effect in schools and elsewhere.'[39]

The MRC found itself rather caught on the hop, with light therapy spreading so rapidly that there was a real risk it would become even more firmly and widely established before the MRC had a chance to adjudicate on its efficacy.[40] Walter Fletcher, the MRC Secretary, bemoaned the fact that the

CBAL was failing to provide any 'carefully controlled clinical observations'[41] and Robert Bourdillon warned the MRC that:

> The subject is… of considerable administrative importance due to its present popular interest. It therefore seems possible that if the Council do not institute further research in the clinical effects of Actinotherapy, they may be placed in an uncomfortable position in two or three years' time….[42]

Fletcher did not feel that the MRC could risk being sidelined in this fashion; he admitted in 1926 that 'the rapid development and popularity of light treatment has found the Committee unprepared to deal with it on the basis of scientific evidence.'[43] The MRC annual report for 1928 deemed only one previously published report worthy of citation, a 'controlled investigation' by Helen Mackay of poor children in London's East End. Mackay, a physician from Queen's Hospital in London, had collaborated with the MRC's statistical committee for her study, which had demonstrated no apparent benefit from light therapy upon children's weight, infections, anaemia or overall wellbeing.[44] The pressing need for further 'scientific evidence' was underlined by Sir George Newman, the Minister of Health, who faced constant requests for costly new light treatment centres and who sought the MRC's guidance as to their value.[45] The researcher who was to provide the evidence that the MRC so urgently sought, was Dora Colebrook.

Dora Challis Colebrook (1884–1965) came rather late to medicine, gaining her MB from the Royal Free Hospital in 1915 and her MD in 1919. After a spell as a gynaecologist at the Jessop Hospital in Sheffield she moved to Cambridge, where she worked for several years as a GP. She then decided upon a career in medical research, and after moving to London embarked on work with the MRC which was to span the rest of her career. She was later to be remembered principally for her work on the bacteriology of puerperal sepsis performed with her brother, the bacteriologist Leonard Colebrook, at Queen Charlotte's Hospital in London.[46]

It was in January 1925, when she had moved to London and was working with light therapy at the North Islington Infant Welfare Centre, that Colebrook first came to Walter Fletcher's attention. Besides her avowed intention to pursue medical research, her family connections helped secure her first research grant; Leonard Hill introduced her to Fletcher as Leonard Colebrook's sister, 'Dr Dora Colebrook, sister of "Coli", is doing some good work under my advice,' and described her 'very striking' results with light therapy, 'eg. very marked increase in weight of some of the marasmic babies concomitant with the light treatment, and some marked increase in milk supply of some of the mothers.' He proposed that she be allocated a personal grant of £100 per year 'in order to secure the publication of interesting results under the Council's name.'[47] In pursuit of this application, in March 1925 Colebrook provided a report of her centre's experience with light therapy between October 1924 and January 1925. At this stage she certainly appears to have been convinced of the therapy's benefits; she reported an 'almost monotonous record of increased liveliness, brightness and vigour, and often of mischievousness in all children' following light therapy, together with an invariable gain in weight and general well-being. Infants who manifested 'general backwardness' showed an 'extraordinarily good response' and the treatment also helped vomiting, rickets, poor appetite, insomnia – one father commented that the effect of light therapy on his sleepless infant was 'too good to be true' – and breastfeeding, the resultant milk supply sometimes actually becoming excessive. She expressed uncertainty about the treatment's value for colds and enlarged neck glands. She suggested a scheme for further research which involved comparing different durations and doses of light to ascertain which were most beneficial – there was no suggestion of evaluating whether the therapy actually worked at all, a matter which she appears to have accepted at this stage as self-evident.[48]

Conscious of the need to evaluate the clinical merits of light therapy and disillusioned by the lack of 'any definite information on points of that kind from Sequira or Gauvain'[49] (the clinicians on his light committee), Fletcher decided to form the new Clinical and Biological sub-committee to the CBAL. The sub-committee was intended specifically to evaluate the therapeutic benefits of light, and Fletcher asked Dora Colebrook to act as its secretary, with Leonard Hill as chairman.[50] This sub-committee was to exist for two years before being merged back into the CBAL and Fletcher promised George Newman, the Health Minister who was pressing him for information on the merits of light therapy, that the new sub-committee would address the issue with a 'definite and more extended programme of work;' 'What makes progress slow,' he warned, 'is the invincible reluctance of clinicians to work systemically or precisely.'[51] Nevertheless, the same clinicians who had proved to be reluctant researchers on the main light committee, Sequira and Gauvain, were members of the new sub-committee. Both were already convinced of the clinical value of light therapy. Gauvain was medical superintendent of the Lord Mayor Treloar Cripples' Hospital treating children afflicted mostly by polio or joint tuberculosis, and both here and in his private practice he made extensive use of artificial and natural sunlight. He had made several visits to the Finsen Institute for light therapy in Copenhagen and, convinced by the results of his own experience, was to remain committed to light therapy for the whole of his life.[52]

Colebrook came up with a proposal for research involving 'some eight to ten workers... half of them, perhaps, to be Clinicians and the rest Biochemists, Pathologists, etc.' who would investigate an imposing range of effects of light therapy including means of measurement of ultraviolet intensity, its effects on blood, comparisons of different lamps and treatment regimes, and comparisons between heat, ultraviolet and X-rays.[53] Fletcher considered that her proposals were too ambitious and imprecise and sent her back to the drawing-board to provide details and costs: 'I think that you will find that your scheme stops short just where the practical difficulties begin.'[54] In May 1926 Colebrook began to devote her energies full-time to the sub-committee, funded by a £500 grant.[55] Like Fletcher, she rapidly became frustrated by the lack of scientific spirit in the clinician members of her sub-committee. She railed to Fletcher against 'distinguished men', 'no-one should join this little band in virtue of his name... men whose reputation covered "fluffy" or fixed ideas would not contribute here.'[56] In July, she confessed that:

> [T]he members of the clinical Sub-Committee appeared to be reluctant to initiate or to supervise any clinical investigations at special centres; the chief difficulty was that all the work that was hitherto done on artificial light treatment... was chiefly empirical. It amounted so much to individual expressions of opinion and was not sufficiently critical or scientific. Further, even the most experienced workers were disinclined to record their impressions in black and white.[57]

Colebrook promised to look for 'reliable workers'[58] for clinical investigation but in fact appears largely to have decided to go it alone in her future work – a decision which was to have a substantial impact on the way her findings were to be received, as discussed below. In November 1926, she presented Fletcher with a proposal for a study of the effects of ultraviolet light on varicose ulcers, in which she would administer the treatment herself, having secured facilities at three local hospitals.[59] At the same time, she proposed an investigation of light therapy on the general wellbeing, brightness, and resistance to minor ailments of schoolchildren,[60] again with herself undertaking the work.[61] Both trials started the following year, 1927, and Colebrook devoted large amounts of her time to supervising and conducting the studies in person.[62]

Eighty-four patients with varicose ulcers received either conventional treatment with paste and dressings, or ultraviolet therapy. Subjects recruited during the first half of the study received light treatment; their progress was compared with that of subjects recruited in the second half, who received paste therapy, a selection method which Colebrook appears to have considered essentially random.[63] Four patients, who had more than one ulcer, received both therapies, different ulcers serving as treatment and 'control'. A further eleven ulcers were only partially treated – Colebrook occluded part of the ulcer with an opaque screen and exposed the remaining portion to ultraviolet light, the screened portion serving as an untreated comparison. She assessed the progress of healing by tracing the margins of each ulcer before and after treatment, and comparing their size. The results were unequivocally negative and indeed suggested that conventional paste treatment was superior to ultraviolet therapy.[64] The results from the schoolchildren's study were equally damning. Colebrook randomly allocated almost three hundred children from a Willesden Council infant school to receive either ultraviolet radiation from a naked arc lamp, irradiation from an identical lamp screened by glass which prevented the passage of ultraviolet, or no treatment at all. She recorded the children's heights, weights, incidence and duration of minor infections such as colds and fevers, school absences, their school progress as documented by their teachers, and her own subjective impression of their wellbeing, together with the impressions of the children's parents and teachers. Once again, she concluded that there was no advantage to light therapy, on the contrary, untreated children even appeared to suffer fewer infections and to gain more weight than those exposed to ultraviolet.[65] Now, it appeared, the Clinical and Biological sub-committee had finally provided Fletcher with the 'scientific evidence' he had sought on light therapy. The majority of doctors and of the public, however, were not to receive these findings well.

Publish and be damned: the response to the MRC's findings

Colebrook undertook her varicose ulcer study during 1927 and her schoolchildren's study between August 1927 and March 1928. She first published the results of her ulcer work in the *Lancet* dated 5 May 1928,[66] with herself as the sole author. A brief summary of both studies followed in the MRC annual report for 1927/8, published in March 1929.[67] A detailed account of both studies subsequently appeared as an MRC special report, 'Irradiation and Health', in September 1929.[68]

The *Lancet* paper attracted little response, although one correspondent suggested that the dose of ultraviolet radiation had been inadequate to achieve any ulcer healing.[69] However, the MRC annual report of the following March was more widely publicised, and attracted widespread opposition, and even frank disbelief. Several critics argued that the results must be flawed because light therapy's effectiveness had already been proven through years of clinical experience. An editorial in the *BMJ* accused the MRC of being 'bent on putting out the lights with a douche of cold water' and expressed scepticism about the results because they were 'at variance with those of a large body of experienced clinicians'.[70] Dr Murray Levick argued in a letter to the journal that the fact that 'all the great hospitals'[71] had invested large sums in light therapy equipment, under the direction of 'distinguished medical men', testified to its efficacy. He concluded that the results obtained in these centres 'more than justified' the use of light therapy. Another correspondent countered Colebrook's conclusions simply by summarising his own experience with light therapy in a number of conditions including tuberculous ulcers, tuberculous arthritis, rickets, debility, and lupus.[72] Another, Dr Stanley Banks, acknowledged the 'scientific value' of the MRC investigations but went on to argue that 'scientific facts may be the truth, but… not necessarily the whole truth'.[73] He summarised his experience in light treatment clinics for children and cited 'the almost unanimous body of opinion in favour of light treatment' to oppose the MRC's conclusions. Even after the publication of the more detailed special report in September, the *BMJ* continued to place its faith in the reputation of light therapy, concluding in an editorial:

> As long as there is a reasonable probability that a remedy may be causally related to benefit that has been known to follow its application, then the medical practitioner is justified in continuing to use it.[74]

The *Lancet* proved to be no more enthusiastic towards the MRC's findings. An editorial argued that the fact that light therapy had become so widespread and had been in use for so long, was proof of its efficacy, 'in the long run neither medical men nor the public can be deceived… if they continue to uphold any form of treatment its scientific value will eventually be established.'[75] The author even employed Colebrook's finding that children subjected to ultraviolet light appeared to have developed more colds than untreated children as evidence that the therapy was at least doing something. A correspondent applauded the attempt to place actinotherapy on a scientific footing but emphasised the place of 'the genuine clinical results already obtained'[76] in this endeavour rather than the MRC's experiments. *The Times* considered that the MRC report amounted to a 'searching criticism'[77] of ultraviolet therapy and Dr King Brown, medical editor of the *British Journal of Actinotherapy and Physiotherapy,* responded in a letter to the newspaper that it was 'inconceivable to suppose that the patient work of thirty-five years can be negatived by a few experiments on a limited scale.'[78] Murray Levick also claimed in *The Times* that the 'thousands of cases published in the leading medical and scientific journals'[79] proved the benefits of light therapy, and another correspondent, John Lynn-Thomas, 'a surgeon (now retired) of long experience'[80] considered that the only cure for Doubting Thomases was for them to visit a light treatment centre and see the 'remarkable, and on the borderline of the unbelievable' results for themselves.

The same argument appealed to the *Daily Telegraph,* in an edition headed on its front page 'Doctors and Light Ray Treatment'. The editorial column railed against the MRC's 'strangely depreciatory references'[81] to light therapy and contended that the fact that the treatment was so widely used and had such a long pedigree, proved its value. This edition devoted a column to actinotherapists' responses to the MRC report; they argued that extensive experience with light therapy in prestigious hospitals had established its usefulness and that the King's physicians would not have chosen to employ it had it been worthless.[82] *The Guardian* agreed, opposing the MRC conclusions with clinicians' experience of light therapy,[83] and published a letter from Stella Churchill arguing on behalf of those 'readers who have just returned well and sunburnt from their summer holidays'[84] that experience had proved the treatment's value.

Some chose to explain away the MRC findings by criticising Colebrook's technique, arguing that the dose of ultraviolet light she administered was insufficient in her ulcer study,[85] of the wrong wavelength,[86] excessive in the children's study,[87] or that her technique was simply 'wrong'.[88] Percy Hall dismissed the MRC and other sceptics by suggesting that bad results would frequently 'be found to have been due to bad technique, wrong apparatus, wrong choice of patient, or lack of skill in the operator; idiosyncrasies also occurred among patients.'[89] Several critics argued that the dose and nature of light therapy should be tailored to the individual patient, and that it was pointless to study the effects of identical treatments applied uniformly to different subjects.[90] Those arguing against Colebrook's findings appeared to be particularly incensed by a remark in the MRC annual report stating that, other than its effects in generating vitamin D, no physiological effect of light had ever been demonstrated apart from a direct irritant effect on the skin, which could equally well be achieved with a (far cheaper) mustard plaster.[91] This remark was echoed in the lay press[92] and the *Daily Telegraph* went on to suggest that 'sarcasm rarely makes a sound scientific argument.'[93] The mustard plaster reference was derided by King Brown[94] and dismissed as 'flippant' by Murray Levick,[95] who suggested that ultraviolet light conveyed as-yet undiscovered therapeutic properties over and above the irritant properties of a mustard plaster.[96] *The Lancet* agreed, refuting the mustard-plaster reference by pointing out that little was known of the mechanism of action of vitamin D, and that although skin inflammation was one physiological effect of light therapy, 'it is surely premature to infer that no others are derived from exposure to artificial sunlight.'[97] Indeed, even Fletcher had queried the accuracy of the comparison with a mustard plaster prior to the publication of the MRC annual report, and Colebrook had promised to verify the statement; her researches appear to have consisted of asking her brother Leonard, who provided a faint endorsement.[98]

Nevertheless, the comparison was abandoned for the subsequent special report, to the satisfaction of the *British Journal of Actinotherapy and Physiotherapy* which was delighted that 'we find here no laborious jests about "mustard plasters".'[99]

The manufacture and sale of light therapy apparatus was a well-established and lucrative enterprise by this time, and unsurprisingly those involved in this venture also weighed in against Colebrook's findings, largely directing their correspondence directly to the MRC. Fletcher was taken aback by 'all this tow-row from the light merchants',[100] prompting Leonard Hill to pen the limerick which heads this chapter. Because of the controversy inspired by the publication of the annual report, Fletcher felt that the more detailed special report should have a judicious and carefully phrased preface which would 'illuminate the position of the Council in this matter, though by indirect reference rather than with any semblance of direct self-defence'[101] and he wrote to Hill and Henry Dale to ask for help in drafting it.[102] The resulting preface appears to attempt to address, in part, some of the criticisms directed at the initial annual report; it commended the scientific virtue of Colebrook's experiments, but warned that her negative results strictly only applied to the particular subjects, medical conditions, and light regimes that she studied and could not necessarily be extrapolated to the role of light therapy in other conditions.[103]

One turbulent woman: the vilification of Dora

Many of the MRC's opponents appear to have adopted a peculiar strategy in this dispute – they identified Dora Colebrook specifically, rather than the MRC or even the CBAL, as their sole opponent. *The Times,*[104] *The Guardian,*[105] *Lancet*[106] and *BMJ*[107] as well as the *British Journal of Actinotherapy and Physiotherapy*[108] identified the studies as entirely Colebrook's work, and King Brown criticised 'experiments carried out by one research worker'[109] and 'Dr Colebrook's Willesden experiments'.[110] An editorial in the *BMJ* emphasised Colebrook's close personal involvement in the conduct of the children's study.[111] Several critics – inaccurately – accused Colebrook of acting alone, unsupported by experts in the field and without the knowledge or approval even of the CBAL. The *British Journal of Actinotherapy and Physiotherapy* claimed that Colebrook's findings had been published 'without reference to the Council's Committee on the Biological Actions of Light'[112] and *The Times* considered that the preface to the special report should have been signed by the CBAL rather than being presented anonymously, to enable the reader to discern whether 'such masters in the field of actinotherapy as Sir Henry Gauvain and Professor Leonard Hill accept these experiments as decisive of the questions at issue.' The editorial identified Colebrook as the sole author of the report and concluded that:

[T]he subject is of such great importance that the public is entitled to further enlightenment from those whose labours in the clinical field have been the means of placing actinotherapy in its present position as an agent of treatment.[113]

Charles Heald suggested that the fact that Colebrook apparently had no endorsement from the CBAL was sufficient to invalidate her conclusions;[114] Heald was a colleague of Colebrook's who had worked with her at the Royal Free Hospital and who had previously defended her findings regarding varicose ulcer therapy,[115] but who was incensed by her conclusions from the children's study.[116] Weinbren commented that Colebrook was 'using a technique of her own'[117] and questioned, 'Why the Council should accept the work of Dr Colebrook, which was carried out in a few months, to the opinion of Sir Henry Gauvain and Mr Duke-Elder.' Percy Hall complained that 'it was not fair to institute experimental examinations of this nature unless the criteria were carefully looked into by experts in the subject… in this connexion no experts had been consulted.'[118] The *British Journal of Actinotherapy and Physiotherapy*, virulent in its criticisms of Colebrook's findings, referred consistently to the MRC special report simply as 'The Colebrook Report'[119] and to her experiments as 'the Colebrook experiments'.[120] In a detailed critique of the 'Colebrook experiments', King Brown laid all the studies' perceived failings directly at Colebrook's door, naming her repeatedly.[121] The *Daily Telegraph* similarly held Colebrook solely responsible for what it considered erroneous conclusions, suggesting that 'the writer had not weighed with sufficient care the effect of some of the epigrammatic phrases in which she indulges.'[122]

Fletcher expressed surprise and dismay at this singling-out of Dora Colebrook for criticism. Speculating about the reasons he even suggested, 'Perhaps the word "Dora" is specially provocative!'[123] He initially put the blame at the door of *The Times* newspaper:

Most of the misunderstanding sprang, I think, from the stupidity of the 'Times' leading article, which made it appear that the whole weight of a supposed attack on light treatment rested on Dora Colebrook's work, who was mentioned by name and in isolation.[124]

In fact, as described above, it appears that *The Times* was far from alone in attributing the conduct of these experiments, and the responsibility for their conclusions, by name and in isolation, to Colebrook. Possibly the critics of the MRC studies considered that by isolating Colebrook they would deprive her of the implicit support of the MRC and its established experts in light therapy; she was, by her own admission, at that time inexperienced in research work.[125]

The fact that Colebrook was female might also have helped her opponents' cause – her gender was obvious in the great majority of articles, where she was given her first name as well as her last, or referred to as 'she', and Fletcher noted that *The Daily Telegraph* even attributed the MRC findings simply to a 'woman writer'.[126] At the time, women were still largely excluded from scientific endeavour and, to a lesser extent, from medicine. Over the latter half of the nineteenth century, male protagonists had developed a number of arguments against the inclusion of women in such spheres, frequently claiming support from some form of scientific rationale. They claimed that women, alongside children and the 'lower races', enjoyed limited physical and mental capacities, reinforcing their opinions with detailed craniological measurements and observations from embryology. Darwin had argued that sexual selection promoted the development of intelligence in the male, who attracted a mate through his wit and intellect, but acted to promote physical attractiveness in women, whose appeal lay in physical beauty. Some even invoked the first law of thermodynamics concerning conservation of energy and suggested that the drains imposed by puberty, menstruation, and childbearing deprived a woman of intellectual energy.[127] Specific arguments against women practising medicine included the inadequacy of women's schooling, women's physical weakness which rendered them unsuitable for the rigours of a medical career, the likely adverse effects of such a career upon a woman's reproductive function and general physical and mental health, and the disruptive effect of co-educational teaching. The paucity of women who were numbered amongst the great scientists and eminent individuals of the world, was adduced as further proof of their intellectual inferiority.[128] Although some of these views, particularly the appeals to embryology and energy conservation, were becoming obsolete by the early twentieth century, there remained a widespread conception of woman as physiologically unsuited for science – though as naturally equipped for clerical, technical, or caring roles, or for marriage and motherhood.[129]

Colebrook defended herself against the suggestion that she was acting in isolation from the CBAL when she braved a debate on actinotherapy in January 1930 at the St Pancras Division of the British Medical Association. The 'debate' appears in fact to have consisted of Colebrook facing universal opposition; she stressed that her plans had been 'passed by the Light Committee of the Medical Research Council'[130] and conceded that light therapy might still have a place in the treatment of *lupus* and some eye diseases, but considered that any general tonic properties were psychological and akin to the tonic properties of a walk in the country or a trip to the cinema. She was certainly intimately connected with the CBAL, being a committee member and also its secretary. *The Times'* complaint that the preface to the MRC's special report might not pass muster from experts such as Leonard Hill now appears misplaced, as Hill was instrumental in writing it.[131] Nevertheless, as I have outlined, it does appear that Colebrook and Fletcher deliberately chose to sideline those committee members such as Gauvain and Sequira who, they saw as reluctant physician-researchers, and this decision could have served to fuel the controversy.

The MRC response – controlled

The MRC's response to these criticisms was generated largely by Fletcher and Hill, who chose largely to employ the rhetoric of 'control'. Both Colebrook's studies utilised comparison subjects, and her children's study would appear to fulfil later criteria for a randomised, controlled trial – her subjects were allocated to treatment or control groups at random, by 'drawing lots'.[132] She also employed untreated comparison groups and subjected her results to statistical analysis. However, Fletcher and Hill demonstrated a wider understanding of the term 'controlled' in order, it appears, to exploit the term's rhetorical impact.

Even prior to the publication of Colebrook's work, Fletcher and his colleagues mentioned the need for 'controlled' experiments in light therapy. In part, this was a call for the use of comparisons – Fletcher was determined that experiments should involve 'large numbers of patients for trial and control, the numbers being large enough for statistical treatment.'[133] Frequently, however, the term appears to have been employed, at least partially, to refer to experiments conducted under the proper scrutiny and regulation of the MRC, and thereby vested with its authority. For example, when Hill originally commended Dora Colebrook to him, Fletcher was initially sceptical of Hill's suggestion that Colebrook's clinic could provide any useful clinical data. Instead, he proposed that the MRC should arrange its own 'carefully controlled clinical observations'.[134] He bemoaned the fact that 'the clinical work hitherto done has not been done under such conditions of measurement and control as to allow well-based conclusions to be drawn.'[135] Members of the CBAL appeared to utilise a similar notion of control as scrutiny when they promised the Ministry of Health 'co-ordinated scientific investigation, subject to proper controls and in which the clinical work was checked and supplemented by pathological findings.'[136] Bourdillon, in his suggested programme of research for the CBAL, implied a similar understanding of the term when he called for 'clinical trials on a large scale under exactly controlled conditions;'[137] he called for the use of comparison subjects but also used the term 'controlled' to refer to proper regulation, 'auxiliary treatment should be exactly controlled.'

The potential rhetorical power of the term 'controlled' appears not to have been lost on Dora Colebrook, who chose to enclose the word in quotation marks when, in November 1926, she prophesied that there would 'shortly be a flood of pseudo-scientific statements about "controlled" experiments'[138] and that these would merely confuse the issue of the effectiveness of light therapy even further. Indeed, Colebrook appears to have made something of a conceptual journey since submitting her initial research proposals, as someone 'quite inexperienced in research work',[139] to Fletcher in March 1926, eliciting Fletcher's rather dismissive response suggesting that her ideas were too imprecise.[140] The following months presumably involved some tuition in research methodology from Fletcher and others at the MRC, and by the time she documented firm proposals for her ulcer and children's studies in November 1926, she appears to have adopted the MRC's prevailing notions of a properly 'controlled' trial. The term was absent from her proposals in March, but prominent in her submission the following November. She considered her own proposed studies 'controlled' partly because of her use of large numbers of subjects allocated at random to counteract potentially confounding variables:

> I realise that in view of all the health factors... which would be quite uncontrollable only large numbers selected at random would give an impression of any value.[141]

The MRC annual report which first announced Colebrook's conclusions employed the term 'controlled' apparently to enhance the authority of her findings, describing her children's study as a 'scientifically controlled trial'[142] and concluding that 'no properly controlled scientific experiments'[143] had been performed which could oppose it. The report concluded that spending further public money on providing artificial light treatment was unjustifiable unless part of the expenditure was directed towards 'properly controlled trials'[144] to justify the expense. The report offered no definition of 'controlled' although the contexts in which it was used and the use of qualifying adjectives – 'scientifically controlled', 'properly controlled' – imply a notion of proper regulation and scrutiny. This rhetoric of 'control' does appear to have impressed a number of critical commentators, who reproduced or addressed the term. *The Times,* although sceptical of the MRC results, admitted that 'the fact cannot be overlooked that it is based on experimental work that has been carefully and strictly controlled.'[145] The *BMJ* agreed that 'the value of such controlled investigations cannot be overestimated'[146] but went on to prefer the clinical impressions of experienced practitioners. The *Lancet* also noted the MRC claim that 'no published controlled experiments'[147] opposed their findings, but again preferred the large body of established medical opinion in favour of light therapy. Controlled work was no longer possible in this field, it argued; the treatment had become so widespread that it had 'escaped from rigid scientific control, and its value can now only be assessed by the long and uncertain method of clinical observation.'[148] The *Daily Telegraph* dedicated a column to allow light therapy enthusiasts to refute the MRC's conclusions. The actinotherapists appeared particularly incensed by the MRC's rhetoric of control; they deemed the MRC's call for controlled trials 'an impertinence'[149] and took 'exception in particular… to the suggestion that hospitals which employ this treatment are wasting public money, and should "demonstrate by properly controlled trials their justification for spending more".'[150]

When the widespread opposition to the findings summarised in March's annual report prompted Fletcher to ask for Hill's help in drafting a carefully-phrased preface to September's full report, the result was a piece which relied heavily upon the rhetoric of the 'controlled trial'. The first sentence alluded to Colebrook's investigation of the effects of light therapy 'under strictly controlled conditions'.[151] Fletcher's preface went on to anticipate further criticism by defending the findings at some length, challenging opponents to refute the MRC conclusions only if they could demonstrate results from their own experiments 'under conditions as critically controlled as those of Dr Colebrook's experiment'[152] and arguing that any claim for success of light therapy should 'be brought to the test of such controlled scientific investigations as that of which Dr Colebrook has here given example.'[153] Such talk of 'controlled conditions', particularly with qualifiers for emphasis – 'strictly controlled', 'critically controlled' – suggests that Fletcher was not simply referring to the presence of comparison subjects, but was using the phrase to imply a properly regulated and well-conducted study. In his preface he associated these 'controlled conditions' with a scientific approach; here as elsewhere he juxtaposed the words, as in 'controlled scientific investigations' and argued that only by testing therapeutic claims in this fashion 'by the rules of scientific method'[154] could they be freed progressively from empiricism.

The MRC's rhetorical strategy appears to have been at least in part successful; few critics attempted to deny the 'controlled' or 'scientific' nature of the MRC investigations, although King Brown argued that Colebrook had undertaken insufficient control of the diverse conditions in the children's homes. He went on to suggest that she had supplied spurious detail, for example concerning the ultraviolet absorbency spectrum of the glass used to shield her lamps, to provide 'a specious appearance of strict scientific value'.[155] Most, however, acknowledged the studies as 'controlled' and 'scientific'. *The Times* did not argue with the scientific merit of the studies, but took exception to Fletcher's assertion that clinical experience must take second place to 'scientific method'[156] in assessing therapeutic value. The *BMJ* was impressed by Colebrook's meticulous methodology, but argued that her conclusions had limited application: 'like all scientific evidence, Dr Colebrook's results supply answers only to the precise questions which she chose to put.'[157] Facing her critics at a British Medical Association meeting, Colebrook again chose to associate the terms 'controlled' and 'scientific', arguing that much evidence in favour of light therapy was 'wanting in scientific quality' and 'not controlled,'[158] in contrast to her own work.

The MRC appears virtually to have monopolised this rhetorical use of the term 'controlled'. Light therapy enthusiasts did cite some previous trials involving comparison subjects, but without referring to them as 'controlled'. The *British Journal of Actinotherapy* provided a glowing endorsement of such a study of the effects of artificial light on coal miners, praising its use of 'controls' as an example of conduct along 'scientific lines'[159] – this study's positive findings in favour of the effects of light therapy on weight, height and chest measurements presumably account for the absence of the searching criticism to which the same journal subjected the MRC report. In another experiment, on the effects of light therapy upon 'under-average, feeble children' in Huddersfield, one group of children received therapy and the other did not; the author claimed that actinotherapy successfully combated anaemia in the irradiated group.[160] However none of these authors chose to describe their study as 'controlled'. Only Weinbren responded directly to the MRC's claim that 'no properly controlled experiments' had supported actinotherapy, by claiming that Gauvain had indeed performed such experiments. Apparently choosing to interpret 'controlled' strictly as meaning the presence of a comparison group, Weinbren mentioned Gauvain's studies of children in hospital wards as evidence of the efficacy of light therapy.[161]

Aftermath: fading light

Light therapy gradually dwindled in popularity throughout the 1930s and 1940s, but remained widespread. Some employers initiated mass ultraviolet irradiation of their workers, in an attempt to improve their general fitness and wellbeing, and the manufacture and sale of light therapy apparatus remained lucrative. During the Second World War, Colebrook repeated her experiments, this time examining the wellbeing of workers allocated at random to receive, or not to receive, regular exposure to ultraviolet. Her findings were analysed by Bradford Hill, who also wrote the preface to her account,[162] published in 1946 as an MRC special report.[163] As before, Colebrook's conclusions were unequivocally negative; as in 1929, they attracted widespread opposition from manufacturers of light therapy equipment, although the medical profession generally appeared less critical this time around. By the 1950s, light therapy enthusiasts were fighting a rearguard action to preserve the credence of most of their claims for therapeutic efficacy,[164] and today the treatment is reserved for a small number of exclusively dermatological conditions in specialist centres.

The 1929 MRC report represented the first serious challenge to the efficacy of light therapy at a time when enthusiasm for the treatment was running high, both among the public and the medical establishment. Opposition to the MRC's findings was swift and vocal, and critics employed a number of rhetorical strategies, including prioritising clinical experience over Colebrook's trial methodology, and belittling Dora Colebrook's experience and ability by singling her out for criticism. The MRC response largely employed the rhetoric of the controlled trial. The term 'controlled' was not defined, but does not appear simply to have indicated the presence of comparison subjects – although the studies in question did employ these – but carried wider implications of authority, reliability, and proper scientific conduct and scrutiny.

Notes

1. Vitaglass was a commercial window glass designed to allow the passage of supposedly health-giving ultraviolet rays. Leonard Hill to Walter Fletcher 4 April 1929, FD1/5054. This reference relates to the National Archive cataloguing system; see note at the start of this volume.
2. *The Times,* 24 November 1928, 12.
3. *The Times,* 29 November 1928, 14.
4. *The Times,* 5 December 1928, 16.
5. *The Times,* 14 December 1928, 14.
6. *The Times,* 17 December 1928, 14.
7. *The Times,* 11 February 1929, 13.
8. *The Times,* 23 April 1929, 16.
9. A. Ness, *et al.,* 'Are We Really Dying for a Tan?', *British Medical Journal,* 319 (1999), 114–16.
10. R.H. Beckett, *Modern Actinotherapy* (London: William Heinemann Medical, 1955), 1–6.
11. *Ibid.,* 1–11; also A. Furniss, *Ultra-Violet Therapy: A Compilation of Papers forming a Review of the Subject* (London: William Heinemann, 1931), 1–4. '*Lupus vulgaris*', or often simply '*lupus,*' referred to cutaneous tuberculosis; although the terms are now obsolete, I use them throughout this chapter with their original meaning.
12. G. Lawrence, 'Tools of the Trade: The Finsen Light', *Lancet,* 359 (2002), 1784.
13. S.E. Dore, 'Uses and Limitations of Ultra-Violet Radiation Therapy', *British Medical Journal,* i (1927), 565.
14. W. Fletcher, 'Memo', 26 April 1926, FD1/5053. Fletcher uses the term 'a

Press "boom"' in relation to the spread of light therapy.

15. Editorial, 'Light and Health', *British Medical Journal*, ii (1925), 525–6; Editorial, 'Photosynthesis and the Origin of Vitamins', *British Medical Journal*, ii (1925), 961.

16. L. Hill, 'Effects of Ultra-Violet Radiation', *British Medical Journal*, i (1926), 617–18.

17. A. Eidinow, 'Actinotherapy', *British Medical Journal*, ii (1925), 71.

18. L. Hill, 'Influence of Sunlight and Artificial Light on Health', *British Medical Journal*, ii (1925), 470–3.

19. See for example, Editorial 'Light and Health', *op. cit.* (note 15); A. Roberts, 'Ultra-Violet Light from Open Arc with Titanium Electrodes', *British Medical Journal*, i (1927), 184–6.

20. J. King, 'Ultra-Violet Rays in Medicine', *British Medical Journal*, ii (1930), 975.

21. Furniss, *op. cit.* (note 11).

22. Roberts, *op. cit.* (note 19).

23. This sentiment was quite widely expressed, for example, Editorial 'Light and Health', *op. cit.* (note 15); Roberts, *op. cit.* (note 19); Dore, *op. cit.* (note 13); G.H.S. Milln, 'Ultra-Violet Ray Therapy', *British Medical Journal*, i (1927), 567.

24. Hill, *op. cit.* (note 18), 472.

25. S.E. Dore, 'The Uses and Limitations of Ultra-Violet Radiation in Dermatology', *British Medical Journal*, ii (1927), 255–7, 257.

26. W.E. Dixon, 'The Therapeutic Value of Light', *British Medical Journal*, ii (1925), 499–500, 500.

27. Hill, *op. cit.* (note 18), 471; J. Brown, 'Influence of Sunlight and Artificial Light on Health', *British Medical Journal*, ii (1925), 477; Editorial, 'The Popular Lecture', *British Medical Journal*, ii (1926), 211.

28. Editorial, 'Artificial Light Clinics in Glasgow', *British Medical Journal*, i (1926), 494–5.

29. P. Hall, 'Debate on Actinotherapy', *British Medical Journal*, i (1930), 149–50.

30. *The Times* special number 'Sunlight and Health', 22 May 1928.

31. See, for example, P. Hall, 'Ultra-Violet Light', *British Medical Journal*, i (1925), 1061; P. Hall, 'Individual Overdosage of Ultra-Violet Rays', *British Medical Journal*, i (1926), 349; R. King Brown, 'Conference on "Light and Heat in Medicine"', *British Medical Journal*, ii (1927), 1194; C.B. Heald, 'Abuses of Light Therapy', *Lancet*, i (1928), 392–3; C. Dalton, 'Ultra-Violet Ray Therapy', *British Medical Journal*, ii (1928), 821; Editorial, 'Sherwood Colliery U-V-R', *British Journal of Actinotherapy*, 3 (1928), 42–3.

32. See, for example, Editorial, 'Light Therapy and Immunity', *British Medical Journal*, i (1928), 362–3; Editorial, 'Actinotherapy: The Need for Control',

British Medical Journal, ii (1928), 661–2.

33. Hall, 'Ultra-Violet Light', *op. cit.* (note 31).

34. Editorial, 'Dangers of Ultra-Violet Light Baths', *British Medical Journal,* i (1925), 708.

35. J. Tonking, 'Individual Overdose of Ultra-Violet Rays', *British Medical Journal,* i (1926), 462.

36. 'Ultra-Violet Ray Apparatus: Student's Death in a Bath', *The Times,* 14 January 1929, 9.

37. Editorial, 'Electrocution from Ultra-Violet Ray Lamp', *British Medical Journal,* i (1929), 163.

38. See, for example, Hall, 'Ultra-Violet Light', *op. cit.* (note 31).

39. Campbell and MacNalty, 1925, 'Report on Artificial Light Therapy,' FD1/5052.

40. Colebrook to Fletcher, 23 March 1926, FD1/5053.

41. Fletcher to Hill, 9 April 1925, FD1/5052.

42. Bourdillon, 'Memo', 21 June 1927, FD1/5054.

43. Fletcher, 'Memo', 26 April 1926, FD1/5053.

44. H.M. Mackay, 'Artificial Light Therapy in Infancy', *Archives of Disease in Childhood,* 2 (1927), 231–46.

45. MacNalty, 'Minutes; Treatment by Artificial Light', 22 January 1926, FD1/5053.

46. L. Colebrook, 'Dora Challis Colebrook', *Lancet,* 2 (1965), 1248; Obituary, 'Dora C. Colebrook', *British Medical Journal,* 1 (1966), 174–5.

47. Hill to Fletcher, 27 January 1925, FD1/5052.

48. Colebrook, 'Report of the Work at the North Islington Infant Welfare Centre Light Department', 3 March 1925, FD1/5052.

49. Fletcher to Hill, 9 April 1925, FD1/5052.

50. Colebrook to Fletcher, 3 June 1925, FD1/5052.

51. Fletcher to Newman, 9 February 1926, FD1/5053.

52. Obituary, 'H. Gauvain', *British Medical Journal,* i (1945), 167.

53. Colebrook to Fletcher, 23 March 1926, FD1/5053.

54. Fletcher to Colebrook, 1 April 1926, FD1/5053.

55. Colebrook to Fletcher, 7 May 1926, FD1/5053.

56. Colebrook to Fletcher, 23 March 1926, FD1/5053.

57. MacNalty 'Artificial Light Treatment. Note of Interview', 3 July 1926, FD1/5053.

58. *Ibid.*

59. Colebrook to Fletcher, 24 November 1926, FD1/5053.

60. Colebrook to Landsborough Thomson, 3 November 1926, FD1/5059.

61. 'Memo: Biological Actions of Light: Proposed Investigation', 17 June 1927, FD1/5059.

62. See, for example, Colebrook describes how she personally kept the children

in the study under 'close supervision' for two or three hours on four afternoons a week; D. Colebrook, *Irradiation and Health* (London: HMSO, 1929), 9.

63. *Ibid.*, 33.

64. *Ibid.*

65. Medical Research Council, *Report of the Medical Research Council for the Year 1927–1928* (London: HMSO, 1929); these conclusions were subsequently retracted as statistically unreliable in the later, more detailed special report; Colebrook, *op. cit.* (note 62).

66. D. Colebrook, 'Varicose Ulcers: A Comparison of Treatment by Ultra-Violet Light and Unna's Paste Dressings', *Lancet*, i (1928), 904–7.

67. Medical Research Council, *op. cit.* (note 65).

68. Colebrook, *op. cit.* (note 62).

69. M. Weinbren, 'Varicose Ulcers: Ultra-Violet Light and Unna's Paste Dressings', *Lancet*, i (1928), 1302.

70. Editorial, 'Actinotherapy', *British Medical Journal*, i (1929), 562–3.

71. G. Murray Levick, 'The Therapeutic Value of Ultra-Violet Light', *British Medical Journal*, i (1929), 620.

72. N. Gray Hill, 'The Therapeutic Value of Ultra-Violet Light', British Medical Journal, i (1929), 620.

73. H.S. Banks, 'Therapeutic Value of Ultra-Violet Light', *British Medical Journal*, i (1929), 662.

74. Editorial, 'Therapeutic Effects of Ultra-Violet Irradiation', *British Medical Journal*, ii (1929), 585–6, 585.

75. Editorial, 'Sun-Worship', *Lancet*, i (1929), 615–16.

76. M. Weinbren, 'The Uses of Ultra-Violet Light', *Lancet*, i (1929), 685.

77. 'Medical Research', *The Times*, 15 March 1929, 17.

78. R. King Brown, 'Artificial Light Treatment', *The Times*, 16 March 1929, 13.

79. G. Murray Levick, 'Artificial Light Therapy', *The Times*, 18 March 1929, 15.

80. J. Lynn-Thomas, 'Artificial Light: Treatment of Rickets', *The Times*, 20 March 1929, 12.

81. 'Light-Ray Treatment', *Daily Telegraph*, 16 March 1929, 10.

82. 'Doctors' Views on Ray Treatment', *Daily Telegraph*, 16 March 1929, 11–12.

83. 'Artificial Light Warning', *The Guardian*, 15 March 1929, 17.

84. S. Churchill, 'Treatment by Light', *The Guardian*, 30 September 1929, 18.

85. Weinbren, *op. cit.* (note 76).

86. Fletcher to Hill, 4 April 1929, FD1/5054.

87. R. King Brown, 'A Critical Review of the Colebrook Report in Irradiation of School Children', *British Journal of Actinotherapy and Physiotherapy*, 4 (1929), 168–70, 169.

88. 'Doctors' Views on Ray Treatment', *DailyTelegraph*, 16 March 1929, 11.

89. Hall, *op. cit.* (note 29).

90. Murray Levick, *op. cit.* (note 79); King Brown, *op. cit.* (note 87); Hall, *op. cit.* (note 29).
91. Medical Research Council, *op. cit.* (note 65), 15.
92. 'Medical Research Council's Annual Report', *The Times,* 15 March 1929, 10; 'Doctors' Views on Ray Treatment', *Daily Telegraph,* 16 March 1929, 10–11.
93. 'Light-Ray Treatment', *Daily Telegraph,* 16 March 1929, 10.
94. King Brown, *op. cit.* (note 78).
95. Murray Levick, *op. cit.* (note 79).
96. Murray Levick, *op. cit.* (note 71).
97. Editorial, *op. cit.* (note 75).
98. Colebrook to Fletcher, 11 January 1929 and 19 February 1929, FD1/5054.
99. Editorial, 'The Colebrook Report', *British Journal of Actinotherapy and Physiotherapy,* 4 (1929), 134.
100. Fletcher to Hill, 4 April 1929, FD1/5054.
101. Fletcher to Hill, 4 April 1929, FD1/5054.
102. Fletcher to Hill, 4 April 1929, FD1/5054.
103. Medical Research Council, *op. cit.* (note 65).
104. 'Medical Research', *The Times,* 15 March 1929, 17; 'Light Treatment and Health', *The Times,* 20 September 1929, 16.
105. 'Artificial Light Warning', *The Guardian,* 15 March 1929, 17.
106. Editorial, *op. cit.* (note 75).
107. Editorial, *op. cit.* (note 70).
108. Editorial, *op. cit.* (note 99).
109. King Brown, *op. cit.* (note 78).
110. R. King Brown, 'Treatment by Light', *The Times,* 24 September 1929, 13.
111. Editorial, *op. cit.* (note 74), 585.
112. Editorial, 'The M.R.C. Report, 1928–29', *British Journal of Actinotherapy and Physiotherapy,* 5 (1930), 1–2; also Editorial, *op. cit.* (note 99).
113. 'Treatment by Light', *The Times,* 20 September 1929, 15.
114. C.B. Heald, 'Therapeutic Value of Ultra-Violet Light', *British Medical Journal,* i (1929), 744.
115. Heald, *op. cit.* (note 31).
116. Heald, *op. cit.* (note 114).
117. Weinbren, *op. cit.* (note 76).
118. Hall, *op. cit.* (note 29), 150.
119. Editorial, *op. cit.* (note 99).
120. *Ibid.*
121. King Brown, *op. cit.* (note 87).
122. 'Light-Ray Treatment', *Daily Telegraph,* 16 March 1929, 10.
123. Fletcher to Hill, 4 April 1929, FD1/5054. DORA was an acronym for the unpopular Defence of the Realm Act, passed in 1914, which allowed the wartime government wide-reaching powers to control dissent, imprison

without trial, commandeer funds for the war effort, ration food, and restrict
access to alcohol.

124. Fletcher to Hill, 4 April 1929, FD1/5054.
125. Colebrook to Fletcher, 23 March 1926, FD1/5053.
126. Fletcher to Hill 4 April 1929, FD1/5054.
127. S. Le-May Sheffield, *Women and Science: Social Impact and Interaction* (Santa Barbara: ABC-Clio, 2004).
128. L.A. Whaley, *Women's History as Scientists: A Guide to the Debates* (Santa Barbara: ABC-Clio, 2003).
129. *Ibid.*, 183–204.
130. D. Colebrook, 'Debate on Actinotherapy', *British Medical Journal*, i (1930), 150.
131. Fletcher to Hill, 4 April 1929, FD1/5054.
132. Colebrook, *op. cit.* (note 62), 9; she does not elaborate on her selection method any further.
133. Fletcher to Hill, 19 June 1925, FD1/5052.
134. Fletcher to Hill, 9 April 1925, FD1/5052.
135. Fletcher, 'Memo: The Organisation of Work upon the Methods and Results of Treatment by Light', 26 April 1926, FD1/5053.
136. 'Minutes: Treatment by Artificial Light', 22 January 1926, FD1/5053.
137. Bourdillon, 'Suggested Programme of Research in Light Treatment', 20 June 1927, FD1/5054.
138. Colebrook to Landsborough Thomson, 3 November 1926, FD1/5059.
139. Colebrook to Fletcher, 23 March 1926, FD1/5053.
140. Fletcher to Colebrook, 1 April 1926, FD1/5053.
141. Colebrook to Landsborough Thomson, 3 November 1926, FD1/5059.
142. Medical Research Council, *op. cit.* (note 65), 14.
143. *Ibid.*, 14.
144. *Ibid.*, 17.
145. 'Medical Research', *The Times*, 15 March 1929, 17.
146. Editorial, *op. cit.* (note 70).
147. Editorial, *op. cit.* (note 75), 615.
148. *Ibid.*, 616.
149. 'Doctors' Views on Ray Treatment', *Daily Telegraph*, 16 March 1929, 11.
150. *Ibid.*, 11.
151. Fletcher's preface to Colebrook, *op. cit.* (note 62), 2.
152. *Ibid.*, 5.
153. *Ibid.*, 5.
154. *Ibid.*, 6.
155. King Brown, *op. cit.* (note 87), 170.
156. 'Treatment by Light', *The Times*, 20 September 1929, 15.
157. Editorial, *op. cit.* (note 74).

158. Colebrook, *op. cit.* (note 130).
159. Editorial, *op. cit.* (note 31). The *British Journal of Actinotherapy* was to change its name to the *British Journal of Actinotherapy and Physiotherapy* the following year.
160. S. Moore, 'Artificial Sunlight Treatment of Feeble Children', *British Medical Journal*, ii (1927), 468.
161. Weinbren, *op. cit.* (note 76).
162. Bradford Hill to Green, 13 November 1945, FD1/4117.
163. D. Colebrook, *Artificial Sunlight in Industry* (London: HMSO, 1946).
164. Beckett, *op. cit.* (note 10), 1–11.

4

Control and the MRC's Evaluation
of Serum Therapy for Pneumonia, 1929–34

'Be damned to Professors – say I – they are apt to scoop the credit and spare the pains!'[1] Richard Armstrong, a consultant physician at St Bartholomew's Hospital (Bart's) in London, pronounced this opinion on his professorial colleagues in December 1930. The matter in hand was an MRC-supervised trial evaluating serum therapy for pneumonia and Armstrong had no doubt that pragmatic working clinicians were better equipped than academic professors to undertake it. His views did not, however, entirely appeal to the MRC, who, halfway through the trial, deemed it inadequately controlled, and re-structured it in order to impose their own central authority over the idiosyncratic behaviour of Armstrong and his fellow trial investigators.

This chapter examines the serum trial and the conflict it engendered between allowing clinical discretion to individual investigators, and the MRC's perceived necessity to impose a centralised methodology. The MRC's decision to 'better control' the study halfway through illuminates the concept of 'control' as the imposition of regulation and restricted working practices over the individual autonomy particularly cherished by some bedside practitioners.

From laboratory to practice: serum therapy in history

Serum therapy had been developed late in the nineteenth century. It enjoyed a wave of popularity in Germany, followed by the rest of Europe and Britain, in the treatment of diphtheria in the 1890s. The therapy appealed particularly to laboratory-orientated physicians, who regarded it as an exemplar of laboratory and animal work which had produced a practical and clinically beneficial therapy. They portrayed it as no mere specific, stumbled upon by accident, but as a therapy arising from the rational application of scientific discoveries. Paul Weindling, in his analysis of the transition of serum therapy from the laboratory to clinical practice in the 1890s, concludes that these laboratory-orientated physicians ranked serum therapy as one of the first triumphs of laboratory medical research.[2] Michael Worboys, in an investigation of vaccine therapy in Britain prior to the First World War, suggests that the emergence of therapeutic, rather than simply diagnostic tools from the laboratory served to enhance the whole prestige of laboratory medicine.[3]

In its commercial form, therapeutic serum was prepared from that reliable creature with a large circulating blood volume, the horse. Animals were repeatedly inoculated with steadily increasing doses of bacteria of choice – initially with organisms which had been killed by heat and centrifuged to concentrate them, then sometimes with live bacteria as the animal developed greater immunity. Injections of live bacteria had the potential to produce more potent serum, but carried a significant risk of overwhelming the horse with a fatal infection.[4] Once the creature had developed maximal natural protection against the infection, usually after some nine months of repeated inoculations, its blood was withdrawn at intervals and serum – the component of blood once cells have been removed – extracted from it.[5] A physician would inject this therapeutic serum intravenously, conveying into the patient's bloodstream the 'immune bodies'[6] it contained which were capable of countering the pathogenic bacteria.

Although serum therapy appeared to be most effective against infections such as diphtheria and tetanus, in which the causative bacterium produced a pathogenic toxin,[7] workers devoted a great deal of time and enthusiasm during the first three decades of the twentieth century to developing serum which offered direct activity against non-toxin-forming bacteria. The potential benefits were enormous and nowhere more so than in the treatment of lobar pneumonia, described in 1929 by David Murray Lyon, Professor of Therapeutics at Edinburgh, and his colleague William Lamb, as 'one of the most serious diseases with which the medical man is called to deal.'[8] Caused by an infection of the lungs and pleura by a streptococcal bacterium – the pneumococcus – the disease classically began abruptly with a fever, shortness of breath, malaise, cough sometimes with bloodstained sputum, pain in the affected portion of the chest, and, frequently, vomiting. After six to ten days the fever would usually abate, often abruptly – the 'crisis'.[9]

Doctors were justified in their respect for the condition – in 1929 around twenty per cent of those who contracted lobar pneumonia died within a few days,[10] and in Britain, it was responsible for the death of one out of every 1,300 of the population every year.[11] By the 1920s, pneumonia had replaced tuberculosis as the second most common cause of death after bronchitis.[12] Older patients were most at risk of dying, the mortality approaching a hundred per cent in the over-seventies,[13] but previously fit young and middle-aged adults also faced considerable danger – which led Lord Dawson in 1931 to lament that:

The way in which it descends with tragic suddenness on men still on the rising tide of their usefulness and with the responsibility of work and family on their shoulders, and in a few brief days destroys them, justifies Osler's designation of pneumonia as the 'Captain of the men of death'.[14]

However, in the same address, Dawson went on to express his optimism that serum therapy was finally about to equip the practitioner with an effective weapon against this appalling infection, just as it had appeared to do against diphtheria.[15]

Serum therapy had first been attempted for lobar pneumonia in 1910.[16] Most British clinicians displayed little inclination to use it during the following two decades; clinical results did not always appear impressive, and administration of serum was considerably complicated by the existence of pneumococcal 'types'.[17] Researchers identified a number of distinct types of pneumococci, according to their *in-vitro* response to contact with different specific antisera. By the 1920s, workers were familiar with four such types. Types 1 and 2 were responsible for the majority of cases of lobar pneumonia, and types 3 and 4 were less common. 'Type 4' was, in fact, a rag-bag of some two dozen different serological types. Serum therapy was available only against types 1 and 2, and each required a specific serum – type 1 serum was considered effective only against type 1 infections, and type 2 serum only against type 2 infections. Prior to the development of concentrated serum, described below, the simultaneous administration of both types of serum was impractical due to the large volumes of drug involved. Serum therapy for pneumonia therefore required laboratory typing of the causative pneumococcus before appropriate treatment could begin. This was a rather laborious procedure, involving the injection of a sample of the patient's sputum – if this was unobtainable, blood or throat washings might do at a pinch – into the peritoneal cavity of a mouse in order to incubate the pneumococcus. After some hours, the mouse's peritoneal fluid was extracted and its reaction to antiserum examined under a microscope. The technique involved the sacrifice of mice and a delay of at least several hours; although a speedier typing method was available, as described below, it was not universally regarded as reliable and was not generally adopted.[18] The use of serum was further complicated by the risk of allergic reactions in the patient, and prior to commencing therapy many practitioners administered a small test dose under the patient's skin, or dropped directly into the eye, to gauge the individual's sensitivity.[19] Others considered this precaution unnecessary, and chose simply to treat allergic reactions as they occurred with injections of adrenaline.[20]

Physicians in the United States were more enthusiastic than their British colleagues about serum therapy for lobar pneumonia and during the late-

1920s, British attitudes started to shift. Recently published American experience had suggested impressive benefits for the treatment and a new concentrated form of the serum appeared to offer considerable advantages over older preparations. The concentrated form, generally known as Felton's serum after its American developer, allowed treatment with smaller, less frequent injections with a lower risk of adverse reactions. It was also polyvalent, incorporating a mixture of serums active against both type 1 and type 2 pneumococcus.[21] The older, monovalent serums were effective against only one type of organism. The new polyvalent serum therefore allowed physicians to start serum therapy at once in lobar pneumonia, without the need to wait for the result of laboratory tests to establish the type of the causative bacteria.

Lord Dawson, then a physician at the London Hospital,[22] recalled that:

> It was a big proposition to have to give 100 c.cm. intravenously every eight hours for the first two days. These objections had in large measure been removed, however, by the introduction of Felton's serum, which was polyvalent to groups 1 and 2, was in a concentrated and refined form, and in the making of which a considerable number of the chances of anaphylaxis were eliminated.[23]

The efficacy of Felton's serum still seemed unproven, however, at least to the majority of British clinicians. The published American experience was extensive, and the results apparently impressive. Stanley Davidson, a bacteriology lecturer at Edinburgh who was shortly to be appointed Professor of Medicine at Aberdeen, was, in 1929, sufficiently moved by one US study[24] to write to his friend and fellow graduate of Trinity College Cambridge, Walter Morley Fletcher, the chairman of the MRC, suggesting that the efficacy of Felton's serum in Britain should be subjected to 'a proper investigation under the direction of the Medical Research Council.'[25] The study that Davidson cited claimed to demonstrate a forty-two per cent reduction in mortality in type 1 pneumonia and a twenty-two per cent reduction for type 2, and concluded that the value of serum was 'proved'. The Americans were convinced by their own work that Felton's serum was effective,[26] but the British were not. British physicians considered that American results were not applicable to Britain, and pointed to the difference between the two populations. In particular, the mortality rate of black Americans with pneumonia was considerably higher than any population in Britain; as serum therapy had been trialled largely on these patients in the US, British physicians argued that the American results might not be generally applicable,[27] and that British trials were necessary because here 'the natural history of pneumonia differed in many respects from that in America, particularly with regard to mortality.'[28]

National pride might also have been at stake. Some physicians looked to the MRC to mount a definitive British evaluation of Felton's serum. Davidson's reaction to persuasive American data was not to advocate serum therapy, but to propose a British study under the direction of the MRC.[29] Some clinicians suggested that the American methodology was inadequate; Richard O'Brien, the director of the Burroughs Wellcome Physiological Research Laboratories, speculated that the American results might not really be as impressive as they appeared on paper,[30] and that he was 'doubtful whether in England the method would pass the sceptical statistician.'[31] Some implied that the evaluation of a remedy also required something more intangible than could be provided in the American literature; Lord Dawson claimed greatly to admire American methods, but he 'always came back to this country feeling that here was a clinical wisdom which is not excelled in any other country in the world.'[32] Richard Armstrong, once he was involved in the serum trial at Bart's, considered that only after published experience from his own country would British physicians be equipped to endorse the remedy, 'The object of the MRC was to have someone in London try the remedy and educate his colleagues in its use.'[33] The British also demonstrated some national pride in their laboratory standardisation of serum concentrations – whereas American workers employed what the British regarded as a crude test of potency, assessing the dose of serum which would protect mice to whom it was administered against one million fatal doses of pneumococcal culture, British workers such as Alexander Fleming and George Petrie pointed with satisfaction to the National Institute of Medical Research's (NIMR) development of an *in-vitro* laboratory assay of potency.[34]

The MRC serum trial

For whatever reason, the MRC accepted the need for a British trial of pneumococcal serum. Davidson had already approached MacLean and Williamson, physicians at St Thomas' Hospital in London, and O'Brien at the Burroughs Wellcome Laboratories. Walter Fletcher sounded out further opinion. Thomas Elliott at UCL suggested that – besides his own unit – St Mary's, St Bart's and the Middlesex hospitals might be persuaded to participate.[35] Murray Lyon was keen to test the serum in the infirmary in Edinburgh,[36] and consultant physician Richard Armstrong enthusiastically committed his patients at St Bart's hospital in London.[37]

A group of physicians[38] at the Royal Infirmary in Glasgow began to conceive a similar trial in their own hospital and obtained a grant from the Scottish branch of the British Red Cross Society for the purpose. Their trial eventually ran simultaneously with the MRC trial and the Glasgow and

MRC results were amalgamated for the final publication in 1934.[39] The Glasgow and MRC trials were, however, quite independent endeavours, separately financed and organised, and the MRC archives suggest that the conduct and progress of the Glasgow trial occupied little of the MRC staff's attention. Indeed, the Glasgow group apparently shunned closer co-operation – the result, Fletcher felt, of 'the sort of jealousy found between Glasgow and Edinburgh.'[40] This analysis will not, therefore, consider the conduct of the Glasgow trial in any detail.

The MRC next undertook a series of negotiations with the US drug company, Lederle, to provide the expensive serum at a concessionary rate. By November 1929, the price had been agreed at 30s per phial, and by December the first patients started to receive treatment. At the same time the British drug firm, Burroughs Wellcome & Co., continued to develop its own capacity to manufacture concentrated serum, which became available to the MRC the following year. By November 1930, the firm had fifteen horses devoted exclusively to the production of its own serum, which was cheaper than the American product, at 12s. 6d. per phial for the first seventy-eight phials then 26s. 6d. thereafter.[41] Further negotiations secured a lower price for Felton's serum from the US firm Parke Davis at fifteen shillings per phial, and from the end of 1931, investigators used all three sera. The sera were not equivalent; the Burroughs Wellcome product was monovalent, and was produced in two different forms, active against either pneumococcus type one or type two. The Felton's serum from both Lederle and Parke Davis was polyvalent, active against both pneumococcal types.

During the winter of 1929/30, Lyon in Edinburgh, Elliott in UCL, and Richard Armstrong at St Bart's, enrolled their patients into the study. Some persuaded their colleagues in the same hospitals to participate too. Cases of lobar pneumonia proved to be far thinner on the ground than anticipated – due, the investigators claimed, to unusually warm winters 'as mild as June.'[42] The study continued throughout the following three winters of 1930/31, 1931/32 and 1932/33. Davidson, appointed in 1930 as regius professor of medicine at Aberdeen, added his patients from December of that year, after a 'hard months' work' spent overcoming 'the extraordinary bitterness that has existed in Aberdeen between Public Health and Voluntary Hospital systems.' Confident of his success in persuading the two systems to co-operate, he predicted that: 'In the future Aberdeen may be a valuable centre for research.'[43] However, the mild winters upset his calculations too, and he was even driven to advertising amongst local GPs for cases to be sent straight into hospital rather than treated at home.[44] University College Hospital (UCH) dropped out in 1931 due to Elliott's ill health.[45] John Ryle, a consultant at Guy's and by that time a member of the recently-formed Therapeutic Trials Committee (see below) suggested in December 1931 that his medical registrar, Reginald Waterfield, be drafted into the study to replace Elliott,[46] but Waterfield does not appear to have contributed any patients.[47] The final report of the study was published simultaneously in the *Lancet* and *British Medical Journal* (*BMJ*) in February 1934.[48]

The study had not run entirely smoothly, as became apparent when responsibility for its conduct passed to the newly formed Therapeutic Trials Committee (TTC). The MRC formed this new standing committee in July 1931, in order to ensure 'properly controlled clinical tests' of promising new remedies.[49] Thomas Elliott was its Chairman, and Francis Green its Secretary. The TTC inherited responsibility for the pneumonia serum trial, and immediately expressed concern over issues of control within the study. At the very first meeting of the TTC:

> It was agreed that a report on the results obtained by the different workers at London, Edinburgh, Glasgow and Aberdeen, with a statement of the methods of control used, should be circulated confidentially to the members of the committee who would be invited to make observations upon it with suggestions for ensuring adequate controls in future work.[50]

John Ryle, a member of the TTC, wrote on behalf of the Committee to Green, of the need for 'better controlled work'[51] and Green responded by calling a conference of all clinicians involved in the study on 5 October 1931. The TTC commissioned a report on the progress of the serum trial from Austin Bradford Hill, although Green deemed its conclusions so damning that they were to be kept, not only from public scrutiny, but even from the investigators themselves. Instead they were to be distributed confidentially to members of the TTC. Green justified his decision to Elliott, 'The criticisms of the work to date look more bald on paper than they sounded in conversation, and to send this account of them to the individual workers might re-open old wounds!'[52] Instead, Green and Ryle sent the investigators a document outlining a 'standard scheme of enquiry'[53] to be followed when enrolling patients into the study in future.

Bradford Hill's report upon the progress, to date, of the serum trial, appears to have subsequently been mislaid. Joan Austoker inspected it at MRC headquarters in the course of her research during the 1980s,[54] but it has since proved untraceable and is not included in the relevant MRC files currently held at the National Archive. Iain Chalmers considers that this document 'likely occupies a key place in the history of controlled trials'[55] and has expressed his frustration at its loss. Describing the document, Austoker and Bryder state that Bradford Hill 'noted in a detailed criticism of the provision of controls for this trial that a greater effort should be taken that the division of cases really did ensure a random selection.'[56] Several historians have considered that the preparation of this report was important in forming Bradford Hill's subsequent opinions regarding the random selection of comparison subjects. Chalmers considers that experience of the serum trial was highly influential upon Bradford Hill's later therapeutic trial designs, particularly with regard to the necessity for large numbers of subjects and for allocation to control or treatment groups at random, and in a fashion which was concealed from the investigators. Chalmers concludes that the random allocation of subjects employed in the MRC's streptomycin and whooping cough trials was a direct consequence of lessons which Bradford Hill drew from his encounter with the serum trial.

Lock considers that the serum trial provoked in Bradford Hill 'a determined effort to improve matters'[57] with regard to the design of subsequent trials. Ben Toth regards it as highly influential upon Bradford Hill's notions of trial design, particularly with regard to randomisation.[58] Desiree Cox regards the serum trial as significant in giving rise to a standardised TTC trial methodology; prior to the TTC's involvement, she argues, the trial had been organised in a piecemeal fashion and serum distributed 'in dribs and drabs'[59] for physicians to test in their own idiosyncratic ways. She also notes that the term 'control' also took on idiosyncratic meanings in the hands of the physicians involved in the trial.[60]

Despite the loss of Bradford Hill's critique of the serum trial, it is possible to infer much of its content from associated MRC correspondence, Austoker and Bryder's analysis, and from the 'standard scheme of inquiry' which the TTC produced to regulate future work in the trial. The TTC's expressed concern over inadequate 'control' did not simply refer to the absence of an untreated control group. All investigators had employed a control group from the start and none seriously questioned its desirability.[61] The TTC did express disquiet over the nature and method of recruitment of untreated 'control' subjects,[62] but its concerns about the study clearly extended beyond this. The 'standard scheme of enquiry' which the TTC proposed to instigate, addressed a number of issues; primarily, the problems which it identified concerned a lack of centralised control over the activities of investigators. The TTC had been formed in order to ensure 'properly controlled clinical tests'[63] and at its inception, the serum trial had been 'placed under the control of that committee.'[64] To the TTC, such 'control', in the context of the serum trial, implied centralised regulation. In order to achieve this regulation, the TTC imposed its 'standard scheme of enquiry' in order to ensure that in future, workers would be 'testing the method on approximately parallel lines.'[65] Ben Toth has noted this interpretation of the TTC's 'control' of the serum trial and considers that the TTC's imposition of standardised methodology, such as the recruitment of comparison subjects by strict alternation, 'may have seemed to the MRC to be part of the overall process of establishing control over the research groups.'[66] Desiree Cox also describes the TTC as imposing order and control over a trial which had hitherto been conducted 'in a piece-meal fashion'[67] and mentions the use, by statisticians associated with the trial, of the term 'controls' as a rhetorical device to augment their own influence on trial design and conduct.[68]

The problem that the TTC perceived, was that individual investigators were each ploughing their own furrow – with results which were in some cases damaging to the serum trial, and even to the reputation of the MRC. Investigators in different centres had their own criteria for determining which patients to recruit into the study and for allocating patients to control or treatment groups. They adopted different treatment regimes and different measurements of treatment outcome. When the study was first conceived in 1929, the investigators had clearly anticipated, and had been allowed, a considerable degree of discretion in the manner in which they conducted it. The MRC's role was to bring together interested parties who could co-operate, rather than to prescribe research methods. The investigators were either self-selected, such as Davidson and Lyon, who volunteered their co-operation, or drawn from the ranks of those deemed trustworthy by Fletcher, such as Elliott and O'Brien.[69]

The MRC had made little attempt to impose any restrictions or regulations upon the investigators. When Green, on behalf of the MRC, accepted Lyon into the study in December 1929, he wrote to the Edinburgh professor asking for 'some information on the methods you propose to adopt.'[70] He wanted to know, in particular, whether Lyon intended to exclude severely ill patients, or those with complications such as alcoholism or nephritis; whether he intended to use alternate patients as controls; his proposed schedule for dosage and administration of the serum, and whether he intended to treat patients with bacteraemia[71] in a different manner to those without. There was no suggestion that Green was attempting to impose any of these options. The choice rested with Lyon; Green simply wanted to know, for the record, how Lyon had chosen to proceed, and appeared satisfied by Lyon's brief reply.[72] When Green recruited Armstrong and Fraser at Bart's he offered similar latitude, leaving the details of the study to them and requesting simply that they 'communicate with us as to their scheme of investigation and their probable serum requirements'[73] once they had decided how to proceed. Similarly, Davidson, in Edinburgh, initially merely sought the MRC's 'co-operation' in a study, the detailed running of which would be left up to the individual investigators,[74] and when he signalled his desire to join the study following his move to Aberdeen, he was welcomed on board with no further instructions on how to proceed.[75]

The result was an idiosyncratic variety of methods and techniques. Armstrong, for example, had developed his own method of rapid typing of the pneumococcus,[76] which enabled him to start treatment with the appropriate monovalent serum within four to six hours of admission. Other workers used polyvalent (Felton's) serum throughout, or changed to monovalent (Burroughs Wellcome & Co.) serum once typing results were available, after using Felton's serum for a couple of days. The choice of typing methods, or whether to use monovalent or polyvalent serum, appears to have been largely at the investigator's discretion. Davidson even considered switching from one typing method to another part-way through the trial.[77]

Most physicians agreed that serum was most effective if administered early in the illness, ideally within the first forty-eight hours,[78] but there was no consensus regarding the point after which it was too late to recruit patients into the study. Investigators adopted an ill-defined cut-off point,[79] or an arbitrary limit of five, six, or seven days. Some recruited children as well as adults,[80] there was no agreed upper age limit, and no consensus as to whether chronically unwell or alcoholic patients should be recruited. Some investigators adopted their own scheme for dosage and time of administration of the serum, and others followed the published American recommendations. Most investigators recruited pneumonia cases of any severity, although some preferred to restrict study to patients who were more seriously ill, such as those with positive blood culture results.[81] Some modified their methodology as the trial went on; the Edinburgh group, for example, decided to switch from treating all pneumonia patients, to administering serum only to severely-affected patients, as discussed below, this decision proved disastrous as it skewed their control group. Different outcome measures were also adopted; although the study was originally intended to investigate mortality rates, disappointing early results from Lyon[82] led other investigators to adopt other measures besides mortality, including white blood cell counts, blood culture results, and recovery time.[83]

Most damaging of all was the idiosyncratic means by which patients were allocated to treatment or control groups. The majority of investigators adopted some form of alternation – that is, alternate patients were allocated, on admission, to serum or control groups. Some clinicians allocated patients *before* typing their infection, resulting in an unpredictable representation of pneumococcal types in their control and treatment groups, whereas others allocated *after* typing, ensuring roughly equal numbers of each type in each group.[84] The allocation procedure in Edinburgh was more idiosyncratic still, and as described below, it was to prove disastrous.

The MRC was first alerted to the fact that all was not well when two sets of its investigators independently published their results. The Edinburgh group described its findings in the *Lancet* in December 1930,[85] and Armstrong in London published in the *BMJ* in April and May 1931.[86] Each report specifically mentioned the workers' MRC affiliations – and each fell embarrassingly short of the MRC's expectations.

The Edinburgh report had initially been well received; Lord Dawson commended its 'thoroughness and balanced judgement'[87] and a *Lancet* editorial was upbeat in summarising its findings: 'In Edinburgh Felton's serum was given to every second case of lobar pneumonia... comparison with the alternate controls suggests that it is definitely remedial in types I and II.'[88] However, Elliott rapidly condemned the Edinburgh report as worthless. Contrary to the *Lancet* editorialist's understanding, patients had not been allocated to receive serum, or to function as controls, alternately. Instead, patients with a poorer prognosis – those aged over sixty, and those moribund on admission to hospital – had frequently been allocated to the control group, for fear of wasting precious serum on them. The control and treatment groups were therefore not comparable, and the results impossible to interpret. Elliott concluded that 'the Edinburgh mortality figures as published were fallacious'[89] and Green agreed that this mishap 'goes far to vitiate the Edinburgh, and the total, mortality figures as circulated.'[90]

Lyon was regarded as something of an outsider by his fellow investigators. He had not found it easy to become accepted into 'the climate of senior physicians', a fact attributed by his obituarist to his relative youth – thirty-five – at the time of his appointment to the chair of therapeutics. Indeed, some colleagues displayed suspicion or 'undisguised reluctance' towards him.[91] The son of a vetinary surgeon, educated in Edinburgh at George Watson's College and at the university, he did not share the Cambridge background which was common to Fletcher, Elliott, Davidson, Armstrong, and Fraser. Fletcher frankly considered him unfit for his position, indeed felt that he formed an obstacle to effective research at Edinburgh,[92] and had maintained a sustained campaign to have him removed from his post.[93] It is perhaps not surprising that Elliott was so uncompromising in his condemnation of the Edinburgh figures.

There followed two publications from Richard Armstrong and his chief assistant at Bart's, Reginald Sleigh Johnson. Armstrong was forty-five at the time, a powerful personality and bon viveur, an enthusiastic collector of butterflies and breeder of pigeons, who enjoyed driving his exotic French car with 'characteristic panache'.[94] He clearly cherished his individuality as a clinician, 'I prefer to sail under my own colours which, as you know well, are those of a private craft or free-lance....'[95] In lengthy, hand-written letters he described in equal measure his enthusiasm for the serum trial, and his disdain for bureaucracy. He had little truck with regulation and administration; in negotiating with the London County Council to recruit more hospitals into the study,[96] he characteristically stressed his desire to 'avoid official correspondence of a nature which might entail administrative recognition.'[97]

Armstrong's opinion of medical professors is reproduced at the head of this chapter. The butt of his remarks was Francis Fraser, Professor of Medicine at Bart's and a member of the newly-formed TTC. When Fraser initially sought Armstrong's co-operation in the trial he sought to contain the latter's maverick tendencies by 'suggesting that A. [*sic*] should work in closer touch with the Medical Unit – if possible in its laboratory.'[98] Armstrong, however, had other ideas. He was convinced that experienced jobbing clinicians rather than academic practitioners were best equipped to evaluate serum therapy, 'the pneumonia work... is a hospital not a professorial affair,'[99] he maintained: 'My message is to the practising physician rather than to the professors.'[100] Fraser, on the other hand, regarded his professorial medical unit, backed by sound laboratory work, as the proper base for scientific investigation within his hospital.[101]

Armstrong's view of himself as a champion of the ordinary jobbing practitioner is exemplified by a characteristic spat over the applicability of his technique for rapid pneumococcal typing to general practice. In January 1932, Armstrong described a refinement of his rapid-typing method[102] which was even speedier than before and which no longer required the sacrifice of a mouse. The new technique required the operator to mix sputum samples directly with diagnostic serum on a glass slide, and examine the resultant reaction under a microscope. Because the method required no animal inoculation or 'special knowledge of bacteriological technique,' Armstrong concluded that 'the objection now disappears that pneumococcal type cannot be decided in general practice.'[103] William Logan and John Telfer Smeall, bacteriologists at Edinburgh Royal Infirmary, agreed that the technique appeared accurate but cautioned that it could only properly be performed in a laboratory by an experienced bacteriologist: 'It requires some bacteriological experience, and would be quite unsuitable for use in a side-room.'[104] Armstrong defended the use of his test under 'field conditions' and suggested that 'the diffidence of the Scottish workers may be due to the fact that the sputa examined by them have not always been freshly collected.'[105] The two Scots roundly defended the freshness of their sputum specimens, and pointed out a number of potential pitfalls in the rapid typing technique for an inexperienced and inadequately equipped practitioner;[106] Armstrong remained unrepentant that his method was suitable for general practice.[107]

In common with the other investigators in the MRC's serum trial, Armstrong had largely been left to his own devices in investigating the effects of serum therapy upon his patients. But his idiosyncrasy rocked the boat in April and May 1931. Without seeking approval from the MRC, Armstrong and Johnson published two articles concerning their experiences with serum therapy; both were to prove an embarrassment for the MRC. The first[108] detailed a single case history, of a 19-year-old man admitted to hospital with severe abdominal pain. Emergency surgery revealed no obvious cause, and the following day his physicians diagnosed lobar pneumonia. After receiving serum therapy the patient initially appeared to recover, then suddenly collapsed and died. Despite this setback Armstrong concluded, from the patient's initial favourable response and from the absence of lung consolidation on post-mortem examination, that 'this remarkable case appears to us to afford unassailable evidence in favour of the use of concentrated pneumococcal serum early in pneumonia.'[109]

Subsequent correspondence, published in the *BMJ*, came close to ridicule. Armstrong's claims were described as 'amazing,'[110] 'unjustifiable... misleading',[111] and one writer[112] even suggested that the diagnosis of lobar pneumonia had been wrong in the first place. Elliott was not impressed, either. He told Fletcher that the paper made him 'very uncomfortable' and noted that 'that feeling was at once reflected in the minds of several people who wrote letters next week to the *BMJ*.'[113]

Armstrong and Johnson's second paper appeared the following month.[114] This was an analysis of twenty-six pneumonia cases treated with serum, with the physicians' subjective impression of the numbers whose pneumonia was 'aborted', 'improved', or 'uninfluenced' by serum therapy. There was also a description of patients' typical responses to serum administration. Although Armstrong mentioned the presence of fifteen untreated controls he gave no further details regarding their clinical progress and did not compare his treated cases to them.

Armstrong considered that the best tool to determine the success of therapy, was the physician's acumen, not the mere documentation of clinical minutiae: 'Success or failure in the serum treatment of lobar pneumonia is to be gauged by the patient's improved general state... rather than by slavish concentration on minor vagaries in his temperature.'[115] His conclusion was uncompromising in its endorsement of serum therapy: 'Unquestionably lives are saved, the patient's sufferings are relieved, and the acute anxiety of his relatives is consequently soothed.'[116] He entertained no doubt that doctors should routinely employ the therapy: 'To those who are interested, we offer the advice to apply the remedy to the first suitable case that arises in their practice.'[117]

Elliott was, to say the least, unconvinced. 'Of course he ought to go forward with the investigation,' he wrote to Fletcher, 'But that is a different action from advising every GP that it is his bounden duty at once to use serum for pneumonia.'[118] Were GPs to do so, he suggested, 'much serum would be used fruitlessly.'[119] He was particularly concerned at Armstrong's failure to compare his treated cases with untreated controls:

You break the fundamental rule of showing that you had carefully studied controls. You name 15 untreated cases but tell your reader nothing about them. Yet controls are the touchstone of clinical mediciene, [*sic*] as of all experimental biology. The paper does not appeal to me as being written in the scientific way... [Y]our paper seems to me like a cry of Eureka, without the proof which, was it by Archimedes, was supplied with the discovery.[120]

Armstrong defended his inattention to his control group by repeating his claim that his article was a practical paper for the benefit of 'the practising physician':[121] 'There was never any intention on my part that the paper should be "scientific". It is essentially clinical and written in simple free style for the understanding of the average doctor.'[122] He maintained that 'a practitioner, treating his first case with serum, would find better guidance in my humble notes than in the Edinburgh or Glasgow reports!'[123] Furthermore, he was at pains to point out that he had, in fact, described a control case. He had described one patient whom he had treated with normal horse serum – from a horse which had not previously been immunised against the pneumococcus – in order to ascertain whether it might simply be the ordinary protein component of horse serum itself which was responsible for any therapeutic benefit. He described this case as a 'control' (in quotes) and considered that Elliott 'has scarcely done me justice in overlooking the case specially treated as a "control" with normal horse serum.' He then went on to damn Elliott with faint praise, 'but he is a good fellow.'[124]

Elliott's concept of 'controls' was a series of untreated cases to compare with treated patients, preferably allocated by strict alternation. Armstrong might have felt that his single control case added scientific respectability to his work, but it did not accord with Elliott's expectations; the UCH man remained unimpressed. Others in the MRC appeared to find nothing positive to say about Armstrong's article either. Fraser, Armstrong's professorial colleague at Bart's and shortly to be a member of the new TTC, was not renowned for reticence in speaking up when colleagues produced shoddy research,[125] and had 'only adverse criticism.'[126] Fletcher, too, was unmoved; after their meeting to discuss his publication, Armstrong considered that Fletcher 'had little confidence in my work.'[127]

Back under control: enter the Therapeutic Trials Committee

The serum trial was in danger of becoming a source of humiliation. It had produced no results which were convincing or methodologically acceptable to Fletcher, Elliott, or Green at the MRC. Immediately following these revelations, the TTC was formed in July 1931 and 'the investigation was placed under the control of that committee...'[128] Ryle made suggestions to

Green for 'better controlled work'[129] in future, and Green announced his decision to call a conference of all investigators. The purpose of the conference was to impose a standard scheme for investigators to follow in future and to regulate the unchecked publication of rogue articles. Green therefore suggested that:

> [W]hen we have the assembled criticisms of the Therapeutic Trials Committee, we attempt to draw up a standardised scheme of investigation which we could put before the different workers, at the conference, inviting them all to adopt it...[130]

The conference followed on 5 October 1931. The 'Standard scheme of inquiry' followed on 9 November.[131] It made specific and extensive provisions, in summary:

• that all organisms be typed before, or as soon as possible after commencing therapy;
• that patients should only be recruited if they were aged between twenty and sixty, were admitted within five days of the onset of their illness, and did not die within twenty-four hours of admission;
• that alternate patients be recruited as treatment and control cases;
• that full clinical records be kept – the scheme provided a schedule of symptoms, signs, and pathological tests to be recorded;
• that blood cultures be undertaken wherever possible and always in seriously ill cases;
• that any reports on the work should be submitted to the MRC for approval before publication.

The antecedents of some of these provisions seem clear. Patients who were moribund or aged over sixty were specifically excluded from the trial, and in both cases the scheme specifically prohibited their recruitment into the control group, as well as the treatment group – presumably the result of the disastrously unequal allocation of controls in Edinburgh. The provision that the MRC should vet all articles prior to their publication, is an apparent response to Armstrong's, and the Edinburgh group's, damaging rush into print.

When Reginald Waterfield, at Guy's, was recruited into the trial in December 1931, he wrote to Green with questions concerning the treatment regime and selection of cases.[132] Green's response was quite different to that given two years earlier to Lyon, Davidson, and Armstrong. No longer was the conduct of the trial to be left up to the investigator. Now Green was able to send his new recruit the standard scheme of inquiry; Waterfield 'agreed to adhere to this plan of investigation, so that all the workers in this subject for the Council are testing the method on approximately parallel lines.'[133] Thus the TTC imposed its authority over its capricious bunch of investigators, and under its auspices the serum trial joined its catalogue of 'properly controlled clinical tests'.[134]

A further reason for Fletcher's mind to be concentrated upon the issue of control of the activities of his investigators promptly arose in November 1931. Lord Dawson, the President of the Royal College of Physicians (RCP) had been appointed to the council of the MRC in July of that year, after a period of agonising over whether to accept the post[135] – the spat between him and Fletcher over whether the RCP's clinicians, or the MRC's scientists, were best placed to undertake clinical research was just gathering momentum, as outlined in my first chapter. In November, Dawson attended a meeting of the TTC and, without warning, proposed that the RCP should join the MRC's serum trial. Fletcher was furious; he had been unable to attend this TTC meeting as he had been called to the Colonial Office to discuss 'economy cuts'[136] and he complained to Dawson that he 'could not have guessed that you were bringing up this subject then.'[137] He went on to state that the Royal Colleges had, in the past, been slow to recognise and help the work of the MRC, and that it would be gratifying for the RCP to 'back up' the MRC's activity – but made it clear that his notion of such 'backing up' consisted essentially of the RCP providing money to the MRC.[138]

Dawson's next move was a direct, informal approach to Armstrong. Dawson suggested that Armstrong 'as a Fellow of the College' should undertake serum work for the RCP with assistance from two younger men – Davis, a medical registrar at the Royal Free Hospital, and Johnson, who was already working with Armstrong at Bart's. The RCP would fund these two workers, suggested Dawson, and the serum trial's results should ultimately appear as a joint RCP/MRC publication.[139] Armstrong might have felt flattered by this approach; at any rate, he enthusiastically recommended Dawson's suggestion to Fletcher, whose response was immediate and curt. 'I don't think Lord Dawson sees his way clearly yet, or that the College has framed any definite policy,' he replied. Pointing out that Armstrong's involvement in the MRC's serum trial was 'only one part of a carefully considered scheme in active progress elsewhere,'[140] Fletcher summoned Armstrong to meet him in his office. A month later, Dawson went to a 'fully attended'[141] meeting of the TTC. Fletcher was present, and Elliott in the chair. In what appears to have been something of a set-piece presentation, MRC workers from around the country gave details of their progress so far in the serum trial. Fletcher concluded that 'Dawson was impressed by all this, and saw that we had here an efficient working machine.'[142] Dawson did not raise the issue of RCP/MRC collaboration during the meeting, but spoke with Fletcher afterwards. Fletcher noted with satisfaction that the two men whom Dawson had identified to assist Armstrong, had refused to work with him upon meeting Armstrong and finding that he 'talked down to them so haughtily that they found they could have nothing to do with him.'[143] Other physicians whom Dawson had sounded out, had expressed similar reservations about the maverick Armstrong, and Fletcher made no attempt to hide his gratification:

> Dawson therefore finds himself in the air. His impulsive move towards Armstrong has led to nothing, and I don't see that he has anything else in view... I keep trying to persuade Dawson that his impulsive choice of subject was a mistake and that he should supply himself with some better idea appropriate to the College.[144]

The subject which would be better suited to the College's attention was, Fletcher suggested, an investigation into the benefits of adenotonsillectomy. Fletcher clearly considered himself to have been victorious in this encounter; his strategy was to employ the 'efficient working machine' of the TTC to impress Dawson, and thereby exert control over the selection of personnel who could conduct the serum trial.

The study continued over the winters 1931/32 and 1932/33, and its findings were published in 1934.[145] The trial's whole embarrassing existence prior to its control by the TTC, together with all data from this period, was ignored in the final report; according to the 1934 article the inquiry had merely been proceeding for 'the last three years', ie. since 1931, involving only 'the two winter seasons 1931–2 and 1932–3.'[146]

The extent to which the TTC succeeded in imposing its centralised control over the study remains debatable. Investigators still employed different treatment regimes; Armstrong continued to adopt his rapid typing method, whereas other investigators employed the slower, routine method. Some patients received the appropriate monovalent serum from the start, others received polyvalent serum at first and switched to the appropriate monovalent form once typing results were known. The duration and dose of serum varied, patients receiving from 50,000 to 120,000 units. Glasgow employed patients from different hospitals as control and treatment cases; the other hospitals recruited alternate patients in the same hospital as controls – although in Edinburgh, serum was not employed at all in some wards, resulting in all patients in these wards being recruited as controls and an excess of controls over treated cases. A range of different outcome measures was described.

The treatment did seem to work, albeit with rather modest results. It appeared most beneficial in younger patients aged between twenty and forty: 'Fatality was reduced in the younger patients in this series by roughly half the expected deaths' but serum therapy had 'little or no power to decrease the fatality from Type I or Type II lobar pneumonia in patients over forty, or in the severely ill cases with bacteraemia.' [147] Inexplicably, Davidson's results from Aberdeen appeared far more favourable than any of the other centres, a phenomenon dubbed by Elliott and Green 'The miracle at Aberdeen'. [148] Elliott even made Davidson check that he had not inadvertently selected more seriously ill patients for his control cases, a suggestion which Davidson investigated and refuted, [149] leaving Elliott to conclude that were he to develop lobar pneumonia, he would wish to be in Aberdeen at the time; 'go to Peebles for pleasure: go to Aberdeen if you get pneumonia!' [150]

Even in the interpretation of the study's results, the investigators did not entirely relinquish their cherished individualism. Some had so convinced themselves of the benefits of serum that they expressed surprise at the unspectacular findings in the final report. Armstrong even speculated that chance had led to an uneven distribution of less severely affected patients into the control group, so skewing the results, although this was discounted by analysis of controls from all centres. The study's conclusion ended with a declaration of clinical impression over the stark figures, 'On clinical impressions the workers were all agreed that the appropriate antiserum frequently produces striking symptomatic benefit in cases of Type I and Type II lobar pneumonia...' [151] Elsewhere, investigators had repeatedly asserted this conviction that the serum demonstrated clinical benefits, as measured by their own experience and observations, in the face of unimpressive statistical results. Armstrong and Johnson made this claim in their *BMJ* article in May 1931, explicitly prioritising their 'clinical experience' over 'crude mortality statistics.' [152] The Edinburgh physicians, in their poorly-received 1930 account of their experiences with the serum, noted that: 'There was no doubt in the minds of those who were watching the patients that the antiserum was of considerable benefit in certain cases even although the course of the illness was not shortened,' [153] and went on to illustrate their most impressive successes with case reports. Alexander Fleming and George Petrie similarly noted physicians' 'conviction that an improvement of a kind which was not indicated in the numerical records was evident in many of their serum-treated cases'. [154] These physicians had expected their experience and opinion to rank above number-counting in the assessment of pneumococcal serum. Members of the TTC had other ideas; Elliott, in his criticism of Armstrong's 1931 report, damned it as 'an enthusiastic statement of your personal impressions.... On a small experience you claim more than even the American workers with hundreds of cases...' [155] The TTC, once it took control of the study and received Bradford Hill's devastating critique of its achievements so far, chose rather to attempt to impose a unified methodology, constraining not only the methods used by investigators in their assessment but also the means by which their results were evaluated.

Conclusion: an issue of control

The TTC had inherited a trial which immediately caused it serious concern. Members of the MRC and TTC were uncomfortable at being associated with the recently-published, contentious reports. Some of the trial's apparent flaws related to the use of untreated controls – their inappropriate selection, in the recently-published Edinburgh report, or their simply being ignored, in Armstrong and Johnson's publications. Other flaws related to the degree of clinical freedom afforded to individual investigators and the resultant lack of a co-ordinated system of working. When the trial was 'placed under the control'[156] of the TTC, which had been charged at its formation with undertaking 'properly controlled clinical tests',[157] the TTC's response was to bring the trial under control by imposing a unifying methodology and by banning the publication of any further articles unless these had first been vetted. The TTC rendered the serum trial 'controlled', by regulating the activities of individual clinicians, co-ordinating their activities, and unifying the means of public presentation of their results. The trial came under the TTC's centralised control; it therefore became, in the their understanding of the term, 'controlled'. Lord Dawson's attempt to associate the RCP with the TTC's serum trial through an approach to Armstrong, similarly fell foul of this control when Fletcher deliberately chose to present the TTC to Dawson as an 'efficient working machine' which had no need of, or place for, RCP involvement. Cox[158] mentions the importance to Fletcher and Green, of describing the TTC as an 'efficient working machine' to portray an exclusively British system driven by the ideology of 'fairness'. However, in this instance, the phrase appeared specifically to refer to a control function of the TTC, in restricting outside involvement in the serum trial.

The story of the serum trial is, therefore, largely one of control. The notion of 'controlled' work was for the most part implicit, from the TTC's introductory rubric and its behaviour towards the serum trial, rather than explicit in this affair. The word did crop up, for example in Ryle's plea in 1931 for 'better controlled work'[159] once Bradford Hill had demonstrated the flaws in the work so far. The technical meaning of the term extended beyond a reference to the presence of comparison subjects; the word also conveyed notions of strict laboratory, or quasi-laboratory, regulation. In a 1931 letter to the *BMJ*, responding to O'Brien's call for 'laboratory control of treatment'[160] in serum therapy for lobar pneumonia, George Petrie associated the term 'controlled' with *clinical* evidence, suggesting that a demonstration of the efficacy of serum therapy depended upon 'a structure of carefully controlled clinical evidence which is strongly supported on the experimental side.'[161] O'Brien immediately disagreed. Reclaiming the term for laboratory work, he stressed the need 'to work out under controlled laboratory conditions, in parallel with clinical research...'[162] how best to apply serum.

As I have previously outlined, a number of historians consider the serum study to be a landmark in the development of trial methodology and a major influence on Bradford Hill's notions of trial design. However, the lessons learned were fundamentally related to issues of centralised control. Upon inheriting the study and its attendant embarrassments, the TTC made efforts to bring its idiosyncratic or maverick investigators into line, and hence contain them within the rhetoric of its own 'properly controlled clinical tests'.

Notes

1. Armstrong to Green, 5 December 1930, FD1/2368.
2. P. Weindling, 'From Medical Research to Clinical Practice: Serum Therapy for Diphtheria in the 1890s', in J. Pickstone (ed.), *Medical Innovations in Historical Perspective* (Basingstoke: Macmillan, 1992), 72–83.
3. M. Worboys, 'Vaccine Therapy and Laboratory Medicine in Edwardian Britain', in J. Pickstone (ed.), *Medical Innovations in Historical Perspective* (Basingstoke: Macmillan, 1992), 84–103.
4. A. Fleming and G.F. Petrie, *Recent Advances in Vaccine and Serum Therapy* (Philadelphia: P. Blakiston's Son & Co., 1934), 125.
5. These details of the preparation of therapeutic serum derive from *ibid.*, 125, and F.W. Price, *A Textbook of the Practice of Medicine,* 4th edn (London: H. Milford, Oxford University Press, 1933), 22.
6. Price, *ibid.,* 22.
7. Price, *ibid.,* 30.
8. D.M. Lyon and W.L. Lamb, 'Difficulties in Comparing Methods of Treatment for Lobar Pneumonia', *Edinburgh Medical Journal,* 36 (1929), 79–93, 79.
9. *Ibid.*
10. *Ibid.,* 80.
11. Lord Dawson of Penn, 'The Treatment of Lobar Pneumonia', *Lancet,* i (1931), 625–7.
12. D.C.T Cox-Maksimov, *The Making of the Clinical Trial in Britain, 1910–1945: Expertise, The State and the Public* (PhD thesis: Cambridge University, 1998), 195.
13. Lyon and Lamb, *op. cit.* (note 8), 81.
14. Dawson, *op. cit.* (note 11), 625.
15. *Ibid.,* 625.
16. Glynn and Digby cite Neufeld and Handel in 1910 as the first use of serum in this context. E. Glynn and L. Digby, *Bacteriological and Clinical*

Observations on Pneumonia and Empyemata, with Special Reference to the Pneumococcus and to Serum Treatment. (London: HMSO, 1923). Walter Broadbent claimed in 1931 that he had used an Italian serum with good effect in 1910, and continued to use it for six years until it became ineffective, 'presumably because the type of pneumonia had changed.' W. Broadbent, 'Reports of Societies: The Treatment of Pneumonia', *British Medical Journal,* i (1931), 446–8, 448.

17. Price, *op. cit.* (note 5), 30.

18. F.T. Ford, E.S. Robinson and R. Heffron, *Chemotherapy and Serum Therapy of Pneumonia* (London: Humphrey Milford, Oxford University Press, 1940). A discussion of the reliability of Armstrong's rapid typing method appears in the MRC report of the serum trial, Therapeutic Trials Committee of the MRC, 'The Serum Treatment of Lobar Pneumonia', *British Medical Journal,* i (1934), 241–5; the trial report was also published simultaneously in the *Lancet,* i (1934), 290–5. (Page numbers cited in text, refer to *BMJ* version). Also see below.

19. Dawson, *op. cit.* (note 11).

20. R.R. Armstrong, and R.S. Johnson, 'Homologous Antipneumococcal Serums in the Treatment of Lobar Pneumonia', *British Medical Journal,* i (1931), 931–6.

21. J. Cowan *et al.,* 'Treatment of Lobar Pneumonia by Felton's Serum', *Lancet,* ii (1930), 1387–90, 1387.

22. Later that year (1931) he was to be elected President of the Royal College of Physicians.

23. Lord Dawson of Penn, 'The Treatment of Pneumonia', *British Medical Journal,* i (1931), 446–8; quote 447.

24. The study he cited was W.H. Park, J.G. Bullowa and M.B. Rosenbluth, 'The Treatment of Lobar Pneumonia with Refined Specific Antibacterial Serum', *Journal of the American Medical Association,* 91, 29 (1928), 1503–8.

25. Davidson to Fletcher, 10 April 1929, FD1/2367.

26. See, for example, R. Cecil, 'Serum Treatment of Pneumonia', *British Medical Journal,* ii (1932), 263; R.A. O'Brien, 'The Treatment of Pneumonia', *British Medical Journal,* i (1931), 446–8.

27. O'Brien to Fletcher, 22 April 1929, FD1/2367; the point was reiterated in Armstrong and Johnson, *op. cit.* (note 20), 935.

28. J.A. Ryle, 'Serum Treatment of Pneumonia', *British Medical Journal,* ii (1932), 263.

29. Davidson to Fletcher, 10 April 1929, FD1/2367.

30. Fletcher to O'Brien, 23 May 1928, and O'Brien to Fletcher, 22 April 1929, both in FD1/2367.

31. O'Brien, *op. cit.* (note 26), 448.

32. Dawson, *op. cit.* (note 23), 448.

33. Armstrong to Green, 4 June 1931, FD1/2369.
34. Fleming and Petrie, *op. cit.* (note 4), 126.
35. Elliott to Fletcher, 4 August 1929, FD1/2367.
36. Lyon to Fletcher, 4 October 1929, FD1/2367.
37. Armstrong to Green, 5 December 1930, FD1/2368.
38. Namely John Cowan, R. Cruickshank, D.P. Cuthbertson, John Fleming, and A.W. Harrington; see Cowan *et al.*, *op. cit.* (note 21).
39. Therapeutic Trials Committee, *op. cit.* (note 18).
40. Fletcher to Tidy, 6 February 1932, FD1/2370.
41. Green to Armstrong, 10 November 1931, FD1/2370.
42. Davidson to Green, 22 January 1932, FD1/2370; the paucity of pneumonia cases is repeatedly attributed to mild winters, for example. Lyon to Green, 22 January 1930, FD1/2367; Green to Stewart, 27 February 1930, FD1/2367; Lyon to Green, 15 May 1931, FD1/2369.
43. Davidson to Fletcher, 10 December 1930, FD1/2368.
44. Davidson to Green, 27 June 1932, FD1/2370.
45. Green to Armstrong, 10 November 1931, FD1/2370.
46. *Ibid.*
47. The MRC correspondence includes no results from him, although there is a 1932 note from him regretting that he has been unable to provide any patients for the study so far, Waterfield, 15 January 1932, FD1/2370; nor is he mentioned as a collaborator in the final report (Therapeutic Trials Committee, *op. cit.* (note 18).
48. Therapeutic Trials Committee, *op. cit.* (note 18).
49. Medical Research Council, 'Clinical Trials of New Remedies', *Lancet,* ii (1931), 304.
50. TTC minutes, 8 July 1931, FD1/5319.
51. In Green to Elliott, 21 July 1931, FD1/2369.
52. Green to Elliott, 7 October 1931, FD1/2369.
53. Medical Research Council, 'Serum Treatment of Lobar Pneumonia: Standard Scheme of Inquiry to be Used by the Different Investigators.' 9 November 1931, FD1/2370.
54. J. Austoker and L. Bryder, 'The National Institute for Medical Research and Related Activities of the MRC', in J. Austoker and L. Bryder (eds.), *Historical Perspectives on the Role of the MRC* (Oxford: Oxford University Press, 1989), 35–57. The missing paper is cited as 1487/VI.
55. I. Chalmers, 'MRC Therapeutic Trials Committee's Report on Serum Treatment of Lobar Pneumonia, BMJ 1934', in The James Lind Library: http://www.jameslindlibrary.org/trial_records/20th_Century/1930s/MRC_trials/MRC_trials_commentary.html (4 July 2007).
56. Austoker and Bryder, *op. cit.* (note 54), 47.

57. S. Lock, 'The Randomised Controlled Trial: A British Invention', in G. Lawrence (ed.), *Technologies of Modern Medicine* (London: The Science Museum, 1994), 81–7.

58. B. Toth, *Clinical Trials in British Medicine 1858–1948, with Special Reference to the Development of the Randomised Controlled Trial* (PhD thesis: University of Bristol, 1998), 215.

59. Cox-Maksimov, *op. cit.* (note 12), 198.

60. *Ibid.,* 201; the different notions of 'control' that she mentions are further explored in my first chapter.

61. Although Armstrong did not report the data from his control group when he published his preliminary findings in Armstrong and Johnson, *op. cit.* (note 20), he did nevertheless recruit patients into one. Armstrong also argued against the method of recruitment of controls, by strict alternation, which was proposed in the TTC's standard scheme of enquiry, but did not argue against the desirability of a control group *per se*; Armstrong to Green, 25 September 1931, FD1/2369.

62. This appears to be the ostensible technical meaning of the reference to 'ensuring adequate controls in future work', TTC minutes 8 July 1931, FD1/5319.

63. Medical Research Council, *op. cit.* (note 49).

64. Therapeutic Trials Committee, *op. cit.* (note 18), 241.

65. Green to Hughes, 29 January 1932, FD1/2370.

66. Toth, *op. cit.* (note 58), 201.

67. Cox-Maksimov, *op. cit.* (note 12), 199.

68. *Ibid.,* 204. This rhetorical use is further discussed in my first chapter.

69. O'Brien was not a clinical investigator in the study but devoted his time in the Burroughs Wellcome Laboratories to devising a means to manufacture a British serum.

70. Green to Lyon, 3 December 1929, FD1/2367.

71. Bacteria in the blood, ie. a positive result on blood culture.

72. Lyon to Green, 6 December 1929, FD1/2367; Green replied on 9 December 1929, FD1/2367, thanking Lyon for his 'full information' and arranging the despatch of supplies of serum.

73. Green, 'Memo', 24 January 1930, FD1/2367.

74. Davidson to ?Fletcher, 27 September 1929, FD1/2367 (extract in file).

75. Davidson to Thomson, 6 December 1930, FD1/2368; Thomson to Davidson, 10 December 1930, FD1/2368.

76. R.R. Armstrong, 'A Swift and Simple Method for Deciding Pneumococcal "Type"', *British Medical Journal,* i (1931), 241–5. Armstrong subsequently refined this into an even quicker method, R.R. Armstrong, 'Immediate Pneumococcal Typing', *British Medical Journal,* i (1932), 187–8.

77. Davidson, 26 February 1931, FD1/2368.

78. See for example, Dawson, *op. cit.* (note 23).
79. For example Lyon thought he would be 'probably restricting its use to patients who are seen up to the fifth day.' Lyon to Green, 6 December 1929, FD1/2367.
80. See for example, Armstrong; Armstrong to Green, 17 December 1931, FD1/2370.
81. This was suggested by Green, Lyon to Green, 5 March 1930, FD1/2368; and by Elliott, (extract) 27 November 1930, FD1 /2368.
82. Lyon to Green, 5 March 1930, FD1/2368.
83. All of these were included in the final report, Therapeutic Trials Committee, *op. cit.* (note 18).
84. Armstrong typed prior to allocation; Armstrong to Green, 16 October 1931, FD1/2369. Most others did not use his rapid typing method and typed after allocation, see for example, Davidson; Davidson to Green, 27 June 1932, FD1/2370.
85. Physicians to the Edinburgh Royal Infirmary, 'A Report on Lobar Pneumonia Treated by Concentrated Antiserum', *Lancet,* ii (1930), 1390–4. The Glasgow group also described its findings in the same issue of the *Lancet,* Cowan *et al., op. cit.* (note 21), but had no formal connection to the MRC and made no mention of the MRC so was unlikely to constitute an embarrassment.
86. R.R. Armstrong and R.S. Johnson, 'Concentrated Antipneumococcal Serum in the Treatment of Lobar Pneumonia', *British Medical Journal,* i (1931), 701–2; Armstrong and Johnson, *op. cit.* (note 20).
87. Dawson, *op. cit.* (note 11), 625.
88. Editorial Annotation, 'Serum Treatment of Pneumonia', *Lancet,* i (1930), 30–1.
89. Green to Ryle, 21 July 1931, FD1/2369.
90. *Ibid.*
91. Obituary, 'D. Murray Lyon', *British Medical Journal,* ii (1956), 1309–10.
92. Fletcher to Pearce, 20 January 1928, FD1/1841.
93. C. Lawrence, *Rockefeller Money, the Laboratory, and Medicine in Edinburgh 1919–1930: New Science in an Old Country* (Rochester: University of Rochester Press, 2005). See Chapter 8.
94. Obituary, 'Richard Armstrong', *British Medical Journal,* 2 (1975), 44.
95. Armstrong to Green, 5 December 1930, FD1/2368.
96. He was ultimately successful in drafting in hospitals at Mile End, Bermondsey, and the Victoria Park Chest Hospital.
97. Armstrong to Harkness, November 1931, FD1/2370. Harkness suggested that the words 'of a nature which might entail administrative recognition' should be deleted before Armstrong sent this letter.

98. Green, 'Memo', 24 January 1930, FD1/2367.
99. Armstrong to Green, 5 December 1930, FD1/2368.
100. Armstrong to Fletcher, 29 June 1931, FD1/2369. (This letter is actually dated by Armstrong 29 June 1930, presumably in error; it is date-stamped 1 Jul 1931 on receipt by the MRC, is filed in the appropriate place for 1931 correspondence, and refers to his correspondence with Elliott which occurred earlier in June 1931.)
101. Obituary, 'Sir Francis Fraser', *British Medical Journal*, ii (1964), 950–1.
102. Armstrong, 'Immediate Pneumococcal Typing', *op. cit.* (note 76).
103. *Ibid.*, 188
104. W.R. Logan and J.T. Smeall, 'A Direct Method of Typing Pneumococci', *British Medical Journal*, i (1932), 188–9.
105. R.R. Armstrong, 'Immediate Pneumococcal Typing', *British Medical Journal*, i (1932), 260.
106. W.R. Logan and J.T. Smeall, 'Direct Pneumococcal Typing', *British Medical Journal*, i (1932), 305–6.
107. R.R. Armstrong, 'Direct Pneumococcal Typing', *British Medical Journal*, i (1932), 354–5.
108. Armstrong and Johnson, *op. cit.* (note 86).
109. *Ibid.*, 702.
110. A.H. Smith, 'Concentrated Antipneumococcal Serum in the Treatment of Lobar Pneumonia', *British Medical Journal*, i (1931), 818.
111. J.M. Alston and J.G. McCrie, 'Concentrated Antipneumococcal Serum in the Treatment of Lobar Pneumonia', *British Medical Journal*, i (1931), 817–18.
112. Smith, *op. cit.* (note 110).
113. Elliott to Armstrong, 28 June 1931, FD1/2369.
114. Armstrong and Johnson, *op. cit.* (note 20).
115. *Ibid.*, 933.
116. *Ibid.*, 933.
117. *Ibid.*, 936.
118. Elliott to Fletcher, 30 June 1931, FD1/2369.
119. Elliott to Armstrong, 28 June 1931, FD1/2369.
120. Elliott to Armstrong, 28 June 1931, FD1/2369.
121. Armstrong to Fletcher, 29 June 1931, FD1/2639.
122. Armstrong to Elliott, 29 June 1931, FD1/2369.
123. Armstrong to Green, 4 June 1931, FD1/2369.
124. Armstrong to Fletcher, 29 June 1931, FD1/2639.
125. Obituary, *op. cit.* (note 101).
126. Armstrong to Fletcher, 4 June 1931, FD1/2369.
127. Armstrong to Fletcher, 29 June 1931, FD1/2369.
128. Therapeutic Trials Committee, *op. cit.* (note 18), 241.

129. Green to Elliott, 21 July 1931, FD1/2369.
130. Green to Elliott, 21 July 1931, FD1/2369.
131. 'Standard Scheme of Inquiry', 9 November 1931, FD1/2370.
132. Waterfield to Green, 12 December 1931, FD1/2370.
133. Green to Hughes, 29 January 1932, FD1/2370.
134. Medical Research Council, *op. cit.* (note 49).
135. Dawson to Fletcher, 19 June 1931, FD5/163.
136. Fletcher to Dawson, 4 November 1931, FD5/163.
137. Fletcher to Dawson, 4 November 1931, FD5/163.
138. Fletcher to Dawson, 4 November 1931, FD5/163.
139. Armstrong to Fletcher, 14 December 1931, FD1/2370.
140. Fletcher to Armstrong, 15 December 1931, FD1/2370.
141. Fletcher to Arkwright, 18 January 1932, FD1/2370.
142. Fletcher to Arkwright, 18 January 1932, FD1/2370.
143. Fletcher to Arkwright, 18 January 1932, FD1/2370. One of the prospective workers mentioned was Davis, described here by Fletcher as working at the Middlesex – Armstrong had described him as working at the Royal Free (Armstrong to Fletcher, 14 December 1931, FD1/2370.) Fletcher, in his note, couldn't remember the name of the other worker, 'I think from Guy's' – presumably this was someone other than Johnson, Armstrong's colleague at Barts, who would surely have been unsurprised by meeting Armstrong as he already worked with him. Possibly Fletcher's memory was faulty on detail; nevertheless his sentiments are clear.
144. Fletcher to Arkwright, 18 January 1932, FD1/2370.
145. Therapeutic Trials Committee, *op. cit.* (note 18).
146. *Ibid.,* 241.
147. *Ibid.,* 245.
148. Green to Elliott, 15 November 1933, FD1/2372.
149. Davidson to Thomson, 24 November 1933, FD1/2372.
150. Green to Davidson, 28 November 1933, FD1/2372.
151. Therapeutic Trials Committee, *op. cit.* (note 18), 245.
152. Armstrong and Johnson, *op. cit.* (note 20), 931.
153. Physicians to the Edinburgh Royal Infirmary, *op. cit.* (note 85), 1393.
154. Fleming and Petrie, *op. cit.* (note 4), 118.
155. Elliott to Armstrong, 28 June 1931, FD1/2369.
156. Therapeutic Trials Committee, *op. cit.* (note 18), 241.
157. Medical Research Council, *op. cit.* (note 49).
158. Cox-Maksimov, *op. cit.* (note 12), 185.
159. Green to Elliott, 21 July 1931, FD1/2369.
160. O'Brien, *op. cit.* (note 26).
161. G.F. Petrie, 'Specific Serum Treatment of Lobar Pneumonia in Adults', *British Medical Journal,* i (1931), 557.

162. R.A. O'Brien, 'Specific Serum Treatment of Lobar Pneumonia in Adults', *British Medical Journal*, i (1931), 557–8.

5

Keeping it Controlled:
The MRC's Trials of Immunisation against Influenza

The transport ship *Western Prince* left New York, bound for Liverpool, on 12 December 1940. Transatlantic sea travel was perilous during the early phase of the Second World War; two days after her departure, on 14 December, she was intercepted four hundred miles west of the Orkney Isles by the German U-boat U-96. The *Western Prince* was torpedoed and sank; sixteen seamen lost their lives and 154 were rescued.[1] Consigned to the seabed along with the rest of her cargo were some 100,000 doses of influenza vaccine, which were to have contributed significantly to the MRC's proposed evaluation of the vaccine in a series of large-scale clinical trials. This loss exacerbated an ongoing shortage of vaccine, to which the MRC responded with the rhetoric of its 'controlled' trials.

The MRC has undertaken a number of trials on influenza vaccines throughout the twentieth century. In this chapter I examine the MRC flu vaccine trials conducted before, during, and immediately after the Second World War, and the various notions of the term 'controlled' which the workers utilised as the trials were under development. By the time the MRC's investigators were planning these studies in the late-1930s and 1940s, the term 'controlled' with reference to a therapeutic trial had acquired an almost universal *technical* meaning as referring to the presence of comparison subjects. Examination of the circumstances under which workers chose actually to adopt the term, however, reveals a number of distinct rhetorical functions which they were using it to perform. Whether employed consciously or not, these rhetorical functions had, by now, become embedded in the MRC workers' notions of their work.

The search for an influenza vaccine

Influenza has been endemic and epidemic throughout history. The current name was apparently coined by the Italians during an epidemic in 1504, probably referring to the disease's perceived origin in the influence ('influenza') of the stars.[2] Some sixteen major epidemics or pandemics occurred between 1700 and 1900,[3] but none approached, in extent or effect, the devastating 'great pandemic' of 1918/19. This 'last great plague' struck 500 million people worldwide; estimates of its overall global mortality vary widely but it is likely to have taken some 50 million lives,[4] a substantially greater mortality than was imposed by the First World War. The pandemic killed some 200,000 people in England and Wales,[5] and its effect was rendered even more devastating by the disproportionately high mortality amongst young adults – a reversal of the usual tendency for infants and the elderly to prove most susceptible to complications and death. Christopher Langford[6] has proposed a partial explanation for this phenomenon; he suggests that the elderly had been exposed to a similar virus during the earlier 1847/48 pandemic, as a result of which they had acquired partial immunity to the organism responsible for the 1918 outbreak. A recurrence of a pandemic as lethal as that of 1918/19 was widely feared throughout the first half of the twentieth century; by 1951, influenza was:

> [T]he only disease which in epidemic form has within recent years proved capable in temperate climates of disorganising the life of a community... the only disease which when it has occurred in recent years has markedly raised the total death-rate.[7]

Driven by fears of a devastating recurrence, the decades following the 1918/19 pandemic saw intense research into means of preventing flu, particularly by vaccination.[8]

Richard Pfeiffer in Germany had isolated a bacillus from the lungs of influenza victims in 1892. Initially 'Pfeiffer's bacillus' – later renamed *Haemophilus influenzae* – was considered a candidate for the causative organism of flu, and indeed the US Surgeon General declared it unequivocally to be so in 1918.[9] However, attempts to produce an effective bacterial influenza vaccine enjoyed little success, and in 1928 Richard Shope, at the Rockefeller Institute for Comparative Pathology in Princeton, succeeded in transmitting swine flu to pigs using ultra-filtered respiratory mucus from infected animals. The filtration process removed any bacterium-sized organisms, and Shope concluded that a far smaller, 'filterable virus' particle was responsible for swine flu – and possibly, therefore, for the closely-related human flu.[10]

Three workers at the MRC's National Institute for Medical Research (NIMR) at Mill Hill finally convinced the scientific community of the viral nature of human influenza during a British flu epidemic in 1933. Wilson Smith (1897–1965) had gained his medical qualification in 1923, and turned to bacteriology after spending a couple of years as a GP and a stint as a ship's surgeon. He joined the NIMR as a research assistant in 1927, and was to stay there until being appointed Professor of Bacteriology at Sheffield University in 1939. After the second world war he moved to University College Hospital as Professor of Bacteriology, remaining in post until resigning in 1960.[11] His superior at the NIMR was Patrick Laidlaw (1881–1940), who had been recruited to the NIMR in 1922 from his chair of pathology at Guy's Hospital specifically to work on influenza, and who subsequently was to become Deputy Director of NIMR and head of its Department of Experimental Pathology. Knighted in 1935, he was dogged by poor health since a bout of polio as a child, and died in his sleep in 1940 from a heart attack, aged fifty-nine.[12] The third member of the team was Christopher Andrewes (1896–1988) who joined the MRC's scientific staff in 1927, six years after gaining his medical degree, and subsequently devoted his entire career to virology with the MRC. He helped convince the World Health Organization to set up a world influenza centre after the Second World War, and in 1946 established the Common Cold Research Unit at Salisbury, which he directed for fifteen years. Knighted in 1961, he was a keen though selective music lover, rejecting Bach's compositions as 'just connective tissue'.[13]

Before they could contemplate laboratory experiments into the cause and prevention of human flu, Smith, Andrewes, and Laidlaw required an animal which could reliably be infected with the disease. Initially, they searched in vain, inoculating mice, rats, cats, dogs, chickens, rabbits and guinea pigs with filtered washings from the noses and throats of flu-afflicted humans without inducing so much as a snuffle.[14] When Smith noticed that experimental ferrets at the Wellcome laboratories in London had apparently developed symptoms resembling flu during an influenza outbreak amongst their human handlers, he immediately tried inoculating ferrets with ultra-filtered throat washings from Andrewes, who had just contracted flu – and succeeded in rendering the animals unwell. Additional evidence that the ferrets had indeed contracted human flu arose when one of them extracted revenge with a sneeze into the face of an unfortunate junior researcher, Charles Stuart-Harris (1909–96.) Stuart-Harris promptly contracted flu, and shortly afterwards the researchers elected to anaesthetise their ferrets before handling them, partly in order to prevent a recurrence of similar unpleasantness.[15] The theory that human flu was transmitted by an ultra-filterable virus particle was henceforth considered to be established,[16] although it later transpired that Smith had been lucky; the illness afflicting the ferrets at the Burroughs Wellcome Laboratories actually turned out to be canine distemper, not human flu.[17] During his subsequent career, the unfortunate Stuart-Harris was to prove susceptible to more of the diseases he studied, and managed to contract a number including typhus and typhoid. The son of a Birmingham GP, he was to become the first full-time professor of medicine at Sheffield University in 1946.[18]

British clinical trials of influenza vaccine

In 1934 the NIMR team discovered that mice – cheaper than ferrets – could be induced to develop flu provided that the virus had been cultivated in ferrets first. This discovery offered the realistic possibility of developing an affordable vaccine in reasonable quantity, and the team subsequently developed a flu vaccine composed of lung tissue from infected mice which they administered experimentally to human recipients.[19] In laboratory tests, this mouse-lung vaccine appeared successfully to generate antibodies against the flu virus in the blood of human volunteers, although clinical results were less impressive. In a trial involving the British Army, 678 volunteers were inoculated in December 1936. Eighteen contracted flu, a similar proportion to uninoculated men, and the results were deemed inconclusive. The paucity of cases for study, due to the unseasonably low incidence of flu, was deemed largely to blame for the failure of this trial to demonstrate any effect.[20] A further 483 boys, new recruits to a naval training ship at Shotley, were inoculated immediately before Christmas in 1938; once again, flu proved thin on the ground, but overall the vaccine appeared to offer no protection.[21]

The Americans, however, reported more encouraging results, and this prompted Andrewes, Smith, and Stuart-Harris, in the summer of 1939, to suggest to Sir Edward Mellanby, the MRC Secretary, that he approach the Royal Air Force (RAF) with a view to a trial during the winter of 1940.[22] Sir Victor Richardson, director of the RAF medical services, offered the RAF's co-operation[23] and with Laidlaw, sketched out a scheme in which five hundred cadets at the RAF station at Halton would receive influenza vaccination. Careful records of sickness at the station would be kept, though Laidlaw blocked Richardson's intention to analyse garglings from twenty boys each month – the necessary laboratory tests, he complained, would mean 'too many ferrets'.[24] However, the outbreak of war, and the resultant mobilisation of Andrewes, Smith, and Stuart Harris, meant that the MRC was, in Laidlaw's understated words, 'not in a position to make a vaccine or assist in tests of efficiency,' and the proposed investigation was abandoned.[25]

Nevertheless, the war also provided an imperative to proceed with vaccine trials, owing to the potentially devastating impact of an influenza epidemic upon the fighting ability of troops and the productivity of essential war industries at home. Furthermore, the prospect of producing the dauntingly large quantities of vaccine required to inoculate a substantial proportion of the armed forces, suddenly became more realistic in the summer of 1940. Frank Horsfall, the Director of the Rockefeller Foundation's influenza team in America, described a method of producing a vaccine from chick embryos – cheaper and less laborious than sacrificing mice and ferrets – which might, according to his own results, prove even more effective than the older vaccine.[26] Andrewes proposed immediate tests on the new vaccine, and the building of a centre in Berkshire to enable its production in large quantities, if the NIMR laboratories at Hampstead and Mill Hill should be incapacitated by bombing. His wife should be permitted to accompany him, he pleaded, and could provide technical help in the laboratory.[27]

In the meantime, the Rockefeller Foundation agreed to supply half a million doses of the new vaccine in order to initiate a British inoculation programme, and the first consignment of 76,000 doses arrived in London towards the end of 1940. Immediately afterwards, there followed a warning, from Horsfall at the Rockefeller, that all the vaccine in this consignment contained live virus – not, as was intended, inactive virus which had been killed with formaldehyde. The British tended to regard live vaccines with 'suspicion and even alarm'[28] and the MRC's influenza vaccine sub-committee debated the possible consequences of administering such a live vaccine. Although such vaccines had been used experimentally and apparently without ill effect, one committee member had heard of a researcher who had developed an unknown feverish illness after inoculating himself with live vaccine. Others were concerned about the possibility of developing influenza should the vaccine be accidentally inhaled, or of the live virus being responsible for actually creating an epidemic within crowded air-raid shelters.[29] The vaccine, they concluded, could not be used in its present form, and the fact that it contained live virus should be kept secret.

Other setbacks befell the vaccine supply. The war continued to take its toll with the loss of 100,000 doses in the sinking of the *Western Prince*,[30] described above, and other batches failed British sterility tests. An additional 90,100 doses were held in reserve. Ultimately, 193,900 doses were administered, chiefly to members of the Royal Navy, RAF, the Ministry of Health, and the Post Office, during the winter of 1940/1. All were provided by the Rockefeller Foundation. Unfortunately, by the time the vaccination programme could be rolled out between mid-January and mid-February, the worst of the winter's influenza had already passed and the MRC could draw no conclusions about the vaccine's effectiveness.[31] American results continued to be more encouraging, and Horsfall wrote to the MRC summarising the most recent Rockefeller findings. During the winter of 1940/41 the Americans had administered 6,740 doses of vaccine to inmates of institutions in the Eastern States; the incidence of flu was 4.8%, compared to 7.3% in uninoculated 'controls'.[32] Henry Dale asked Bradford Hill to comment on the statistical significance of these apparently impressive American figures. 'As usual', reported Dale, 'this statistical consideration amounts to a cold-water douche, but not quite so cold as in some cases.'[33] He concluded that the American findings justified a further programme of vaccination for the following winter, but that such a programme 'would have to be regarded as still experimental.'[34]

Thomas Mackie, Professor of Bacteriology at Edinburgh University, offered to help settle the question of vaccine effectiveness with a trial on his students.[35] Mellanby, mindful that 'these Scottish folk are very touchy and are always wanting to receive special treatment... especially when they think that they are being left out in the cold,' asked Andrewes to 'bring him into the picture'[36] in order to discourage such maverick intervention. In December 1941 the MRC team inoculated some 12,000 volunteers in the various Home Commands and left a similar number of uninoculated subjects for comparison; once again, the anticipated flu epidemic failed to materialise, and the vaccine's effectiveness remained uncertain.[37] In 1943, another Scot, Ian Nicoll Sutherland, the Medical Officer for the Scottish Department of Health, offered his help but cautioned that his own trials of influenza vaccine in nurses had proved negative. Discouraged, however, by the equivocal or negative results from the UK and continuing problems with supply, Andrewes recommended no further investigations at present 'as there is no new material ready for trial and the previous results do not justify a mere repetition.'[38]

Once again, American reports of successful vaccine trials prompted a resurgence of interest in the UK. Apparently impressive results in 1944 from a US study of a new concentrated influenza vaccine[39] led Andrewes to suggest a joint MRC, Ministry of Health, and armed forces meeting[40] at which he recommended a mass inoculation programme. The conference agreed that the armed forces and civilian personnel in essential war industries, should receive priority for vaccination and that some six million doses would be required.[41] This time, the Americans were unable to help, all their supplies being earmarked for vaccination of their own troops, and the conference decided to approach laboratories in South Africa, Canada, and Australia. Manufacture in Britain was still unthinkable – with each vaccine dose requiring two eggs for its manufacture, the nation's supply of dehydrated egg, the housewife's staple food, would have been seriously compromised.[42]

The Commonwealth laboratories were able to supply only a fraction of the required six million doses. Some 500,000 doses should be available for the winter of 1944/45 – insufficient for mass vaccination but enough, declared Marinus van den Ende of the NIMR, for a 'further large-scale trial.'[43] Air Marshal Sir Harold Whittingham (1887–1983), Honorary Physician to the King, Director of Hygiene at the Air Ministry, and Chief Executive Officer of the Government's Flying Personnel Research Committee,[44] agreed that the restricted supplies should be reserved for 'adequate well controlled trials'.[45] Vaccine supply proved even slower than anticipated, however, and the first consignment of 1,176 ampoules did not arrive from Australia until February 1945.[46] The MRC had received just 25,000 doses by May 1945 and 50,000 by June. Attention turned towards 'extensive trials… in stable Service or civilian communities' over the forthcoming winter; the 50,000 doses already received would be used for 'controlled trials' in these populations, while a further million doses should be ordered for protective vaccination of personnel in the armed services and Ministry of Health.[47] Stuart-Harris was the obvious candidate to supervise these trials, notwithstanding the fact that he was then stationed in Singapore; with the RAF in his pocket, Air Marshal Whittingham was prepared to whisk him back by air.[48]

Just as the onset of war had disrupted plans for vaccine trials, its ending also threw a spanner in the works. During wartime, researchers had large, stable populations of servicemen and workers to study; now demobilisation, leave, and a variety of individual postings threatened to reduce any large-scale trial to administrative chaos. Smaller trials on more stable populations now seemed more attractive – Andrewes suggested small-scale trials upon prisoners-of-war; Graham Wilson, Professor of Bacteriology at the London School of Hygiene and Tropical medicine and the director of the MRC's Emergency Public Health Laboratory Service, offered the inmates of mental hospitals; William Bradley from the Ministry of Health advocated studies in camps of displaced persons; and Whittingham suggested studying 'small controlled groups' of around two thousand servicemen.[49] Quite what he intended by 'controlled' in this context, I shall discuss below.

Stuart-Harris arrived to supervise the trials on 22 December, despite Whittingham's promise of a speedy transfer, his journey from Singapore had taken eleven days. By the time Mellanby brought him up to speed at a meeting on 1 January 1946, the country was already gripped by an influenza outbreak and deaths were rising. Within two weeks Stuart-Harris had organised vaccine trials amongst students, nurses, and factory workers in Britain and in displaced persons' camps and civilian internee centres in Germany. The trial method was left up to those responsible for running it locally, although Stuart-Harris made 'suggestions', including the use of alternate cases as untreated comparison subjects, which were followed with varying degrees of rigour.[50] Hospitals and local medical officers were asked to participate in a spotting system, submitting blood and garglings from suspected flu sufferers in order to identify local outbreaks at the earliest opportunity. Eventually, 5,729 people in Britain and around 8,500 in Germany, received influenza vaccination, most towards the end of January 1946.

The trial was far from an overwhelming success. In July 1946, Stuart-Harris reported to the MRC that follow-up of cases had proved problematical, particularly given the dilatory attitude of undergraduates, mostly medical students, to bother to report their illnesses on time. Nurses had proved to be far more reliable subjects.[51] Most of the winter's influenza subsequently turned out to have been caused by the B virus strain, recently described by the Americans in 1940, rather than the more common A strain which Smith, Andrewes, and Laidlaw had originally isolated; the vaccine under test contained A virus strains only, and offered no protection against B strains. Doctors proved unreliable in their diagnosis of influenza – difficult to distinguish on clinical grounds from a bad cold – and serological testing of 'spotters' suggested that some forty per cent of those diagnosed with influenza did not have flu at all. Furthermore, the epidemic had proved patchy, affecting only some geographical areas, and did not severely affect any of the populations under study, limiting the scope for the vaccine to produce any demonstrable effect. Most importantly of all, Stuart-Harris concluded, the immunisation programme had started too late in the season to be of significant benefit, large numbers of subjects having already contracted flu before they had the opportunity to be immunised. Some populations did appear to benefit from immunisation – workers at the Woolwich Arsenal, for example, were diagnosed with flu at a rate of 5.08% in inoculated individuals compared with 10.9% in those not inoculated, and students in Glasgow appeared to derive similar benefit – but overall Stuart-Harris had to allow that this was yet another inconclusive study. He suggested a further trial, planned well in advance, with more rigorous procedures for recruiting control cases and for follow-up.[52]

A conference at the MRC in July 1946 agreed to proceed with this trial and to start planning it immediately.[53] Over the following winter the team administered some 20,000 inoculations, between November 1946 and January 1947, to pupils in public and preparatory schools, inmates of mental institutions, conscripts to Army Preliminary Training Centres, and a smaller number of nurses, prisoners-of-war, and patients of GPs. They observed an equal number of uninoculated people for comparison; allocation to the inoculated or uninoculated condition was on an alternate-case basis, or in some instances, predominantly schools, by alternate groups, each school house comprising a group. Once again, the results were deemed disappointing, and by no means approached the considerable success reported by American workers. The team blamed a low incidence of flu, together with another problem which workers were then beginning to appreciate; the antigenic structure of the influenza virus was not stable, but appeared to be subject to change. This implied that new virus strains could arise, against which vaccines prepared from older strains might prove useless.[54]

The first proposal for an influenza vaccine trial comparing the effects of real vaccine with 'dummy' injections containing formalin – responsible for the stinging sensation when the vaccine was administered – and alum, arose at a meeting in January 1949. Some eight thousand staff at Army and RAF hospitals, and inhabitants of the army camp at Catterick, would receive either vaccine or placebo on an alternate-case basis.[55] By now, the British egg supply situation had improved, and Freddy Himmelweit, a German-Jewish pathologist who had moved to Britain before the war, considered that he could manufacture some 2,000 doses weekly. This proposed trial receives no further mention.

By 1951, the question of vaccine efficacy was still unresolved; the MRC's influenza team deemed that their trials to date had proved 'inconclusive'[56] and considered that 'controlled trials of vaccines are still needed and will be for some time.'[57] After small-scale trials in 1950[58] and 1951[59] to assess the serological response to immunisation, they initiated a large trial in 1952, involving industrial workers as well as nurses, servicemen and students. Manufacturing firms were almost universal in offering their co-operation, although GPs proved less amenable – one member of the MRC team concluded that the announcement of the trial in the medical press had rather the appearance of a direction for GPs, and should have politely requested their co-operation instead.[60] A 'special trial',[61] a sub-set of the main trial, involved immunising five hundred workers from Vauxhall Motors in Luton, and visiting at home any who became ill in order to obtain garglings, blood samples, and nasal swabs. One local GP was so incensed at the prospect of his patients being attended uninvited by another practitioner that he threatened legal action should this occur, though most of his colleagues reluctantly accepted the MRC's proposals following a meeting between the MRC and the local branch of the BMA at which the Influenza Vaccine Committee received a critical reception from GPs.[62] Altogether, the MRC doctors made 217 such home visits, although the invalid workers hardly seemed ravaged by their disease – fifty-nine were not even at home when the researchers called, and only fifty-five manifested symptoms and signs which the investigators considered might represent flu. Laboratory analysis of blood, garglings and mucus confirmed this clinical diagnosis in around two-thirds of those suspected of having flu.[63]

As for the main trial, 12,710 individuals received vaccine during the winter of 1952/53 – half received influenza vaccine, and half an older, bacterial, 'anti-catarrhal' vaccine as a control. Once again, the research was dogged by a low prevalence of flu, but nevertheless the study appeared to demonstrate a forty per cent reduction in flu amongst vaccinated subjects compared to controls. The MRC considered that it had demonstrated the first genuinely encouraging British results from a flu vaccination trial.

Clinical trials of influenza vaccines continued, and are ongoing. Current practice is to monitor the possible emergence of new virus strains, in particular from China – the apparent source of most recent epidemic strains[64] – and to formulate a new vaccine each year, appropriate to the predicted flu virus strains.

The rhetoric of control in the flu vaccination trials

All these MRC trials employed comparison 'control' subjects. On occasion, the workers describing the trials used the terms 'controlled trial' or 'controlled experiment'. Although not defined, the ostensible meaning of the term 'controlled' appears to have stabilised, by this period, to refer to a trial with comparison subjects. Thus when the MRC influenza vaccine committee decided, in 1945, to reserve 50,000 vaccine doses for 'controlled trials and to use the remainder without controls'[65] they apparently intended the term 'controlled' to refer to the presence of comparison subjects. Similarly, an editorial in the *BMJ*[66] praised the MRC's large 1952 trial, describing it as 'controlled' in direct contrast to previous, inconclusive trials which had inadequate allocation of untreated subjects. Again, the term 'controlled' appears here to refer specifically to the presence of adequate numbers of untreated individuals for comparison with those receiving treatment. However, on other occasions, the workers referred to the same experiments simply as 'trials', sometimes with another qualifier such as 'field trials', 'large-scale trials' or 'small-scale trials'. There appear to be a number of particular contexts in which they chose to employ the term 'controlled.' These contexts have little to do with simply establishing the presence of comparison subjects, which was in any case hardly necessary by this time – the use of untreated individuals for comparison in clinical flu vaccine trials appears to have been universal, none of the British workers questioned their necessity, and all published studies from Britain and the US employed them. Rather, the word 'controlled' appears in a number of specific instances, predominantly with an extended rhetorical function.

The rhetorical use of the term 'controlled' is further emphasised by its occasional modification by an adverb; for example, 'carefully controlled'[67] or 'well controlled'.[68] These adverbs do not generally appear to refer to the careful selection of comparison subjects, but are employed to enhance other rhetorical effects of the word. Furthermore, in their publications the workers reserved the term 'controlled' almost exclusively for clinical trials. They did not use the term in their numerous papers detailing their laboratory experiments, even though these experiments frequently did employ untreated animals or human subjects for comparison. To choose to describe clinical studies as 'controlled' and not to use the term in relation to laboratory work suggests that the term has a function over and above its description of the presence of comparison subjects.

In this analysis I have examined MRC documents – predominantly intended for internal attention – and the workers' resulting publications in journals such as the *BMJ* and *Lancet,* where the intended readership was presumably the wider community of medical practitioners to whom the rhetoric of 'controlled' trials was directed. The internal documents, however, are generally minutes of meetings attended not only by MRC workers but also by representatives from the armed services as well as government. The MRC was negotiating with government for funds and for the right to exclusive access to flu vaccine supplies, and was negotiating with the armed forces for access to service personnel who could perform and act as subjects for the MRC trials. The rhetoric of control, employed by clinician trialists during these meetings, could well have been intended to bolster the MRC's case for the benefit of these various audiences.

Besides describing 'controlled trials', workers frequently referred simply to 'controls.' This term was used to describe untreated – or 'dummy'-treated – humans or animals, or the sham preparation used for inoculating them. The audience for this particular term appears to be medical; when the MRC group prepared near-identical statements announcing the large 1952 trial to the lay and medical press, they chose to describe their deliberately inefficacious comparison vaccine as a 'control'[69] to their medical audience, and as a 'contrast'[70] to their lay readers. The term 'control' might have been regarded as too technical for public consumption.

There are a number of specific rhetorical contexts in which workers chose to employ the term 'controlled'. In each, the term was at least partially employed to persuade others to a point of view, or to justify a suggestion. In summary, these contexts include the use of the term with reference to the MRC's regulation of vaccine use and supply, particularly in relation to the shortage of vaccine; an ordered, fixed population or conditions for a study; and to establish a study's credentials as having been efficiently designed and executed. I shall consider each in turn.

'Controlled trials' in relation to the MRC's regulation of vaccine supply

Historians have noted instances in which the MRC, faced with a shortage of supplies of a new drug, employed clinical trials as a means of establishing its own authority over drug distribution. Jonathan Liebenau[71] and Desiree Cox[72] have examined the MRC's regulation of insulin supply in the early-1920s, when supplies were short but public demand for the new drug was intense. Liebenau discusses the MRC's reservations concerning whether patent rights alone would allow it to exert sufficient control over the supply of insulin[73] and its use of standardisation and clinical trials to exert a form of moral control over manufacturers and clinicians. Cox argues that the MRC promoted its clinical trials as a morally responsible response to insulin shortage, and its secretary Walter Fletcher portrayed his investigators as 'noble scientists' within this endeavour. Alan Yoshioka makes a related point regarding streptomycin supply in 1946 and 1947 and argues that the MRC employed clinical trials as a means of managing the distribution of the drug while it was scarce. He suggests that the MRC pointed to the shortage of streptomycin to justify not only the design of its trials, particularly with regard to the use of comparison subjects and random allocation of subjects to treatment or comparison groups, but also the type of patients who would be eligible for inclusion, the clinical centres which could participate, and the MRC's claim that it was best qualified to conduct the proper research.[74] Ben Toth[75] similarly suggests that the MRC deliberately emphasised the scarcity, potential toxicity, and uncertain benefit of streptomycin to justify its control of the drug through clinical trials. There are other instances of the same MRC tactic; Yoshioka mentions, for example, that one reason for the creation of the MRC's Penicillin Clinical Trials Committee during the Second World War was to control distribution of this novel and scarce drug.[76]

Similarly, the MRC workers investigating flu vaccine appeared to consider that the MRC was the proper body to regulate its distribution. Although supply was problematical, as outlined above, there does appear to have been substantial demand for vaccine, both from doctors attempting to obtain supplies for their patients,[77] and directly from members of the public.[78] The MRC was characteristically forthright in arguing to establish itself as the appropriate authority to oversee allocation of vaccine supply, and enlisted the rhetoric of the 'controlled trial' to support its case. Frequently, MRC documents associated the need for 'controlled' studies with a shortage of vaccine supply, or with the MRC's credentials as the proper body to regulate supply. The term 'controlled' served to reinforce these credentials. When the press announced in 1945 that 'a large amount of vaccine has been brought over to this country,' Professor Graham Wilson faced requests from practitioners and their patients for supplies 'for general use'. He asked Andrewes for permission to refuse such requests by stating that the vaccine available 'is to be restricted for purposes of controlled investigation.'[79] The original draft of this letter contained the phrase 'control investigation' which has been amended, apparently in Wilson's own hand, to 'controlled investigation'. 'Control investigation' was a term sometimes used specifically to describe a study with comparison controls and Wilson's decision to amend it suggests that he intended 'controlled' to serve an enhanced rhetorical function, conveying more than simply the presence of comparison subjects. Andrewes agreed with his suggestion, noting that: 'The setting aside of

50,000 doses for controlled clinical trials in civilians' had been recorded in the minutes of their previous meeting.[80] This form of rhetoric was subsequently employed to counter requests for vaccine; for example, when a GP, Dr McKnight, wrote asking for vaccine for 'himself and one other' Wilson expressed his regret that 'The Influenza Vaccine Trials Committee is arranging for a controlled investigation this winter of vaccine that will be supplied free of charge, but this will not be distributed to general practitioners.'[81] David Robinson, a bacteriologist working in the Liverpool City Laboratories, received a marginally more encouraging response when he wrote to enquire whether any vaccine could be made available for his staff. Wilson emphasised that vaccine supply was 'restricted to workers who are able to carry out a strictly controlled investigation designed to find out whether the vaccine confers any considerable degree of protection…'[82] but implied that Robinson might be granted access to vaccine supplies if he were in a position to carry out such research; possibly this less than outright refusal was a consequence of Robinson's position as the kind of laboratory-based scientist favoured by the MRC. The MRC's decision in 1951 not to offer routine inoculation to large groups such as the services was also justified because 'controlled trials of vaccines are still needed and will be for some time.'[83]

Problems with vaccine supply prompted a number of calls for 'controlled' investigation, with the MRC workers determining vaccine distribution. When supplies in 1944 fell well short of what had been anticipated, owing to the US government's decision to use all its own vaccine to inoculate the US Army, Whittingham pointed out that the amount of vaccine available in the UK was insufficient for a widespread inoculation programme and suggested withholding vaccine for 'adequate well controlled trials' instead.[84] The following June, only 50,000 doses had been received out of the 600,000 on order, and it was agreed that the doses in hand should be reserved for 'controlled experiments'.[85] Rejecting the suggestion that vaccine should be released for general inoculation of the civilian population, Wilson emphasised that supplies were to be issued only for the purposes of 'a carefully controlled investigation'[86] and Andrewes earmarked the same 50,000 doses for 'carefully controlled trials in civilians'.[87] In a similar use of the term, though not in relation to vaccine supply, members of the MRC influenza conference resisted calls for the issue of face masks to protect against exposure to flu, by promising 'controlled experiments' to determine their efficacy.[88]

The MRC was pointing to its own therapeutic trials as a justification for its position as the determinant of scarce vaccine supply. Its use of the term 'controlled' represented an important rhetorical tactic to reinforce this position.

'Controlled' as 'ordered'

Flu vaccine trials upon shifting or itinerant populations would be impractical; Sir Victor Richardson considered that 'a fixed population... is obviously a primary consideration' when he offered the RAF's services in 1939.[89] The term 'controlled' appears to have been applied, on occasion, to emphasise the necessity of performing trials on adequately stable populations, or under suitably stable conditions. In some instances, the term also appears to have served to justify the MRC's failure to mount adequate studies due to unstable circumstances.

The MRC influenza vaccine conference concluded that 'stable Service or civilian communities' comprised 'suitable communities for controlled experiments'[90] in 1945. It required 'lengthy discussion' to reach this consensus – conceivably the term 'controlled' helped to deliver a useful rhetorical impact. Later that year, when demobilisation and disorder following the cessation of hostilities threatened to scupper any arrangements for organised trials, Andrewes explained that 'no complete arrangements had yet been made for controlled clinical trials in this country'[91] as a result. His use of 'controlled' implied that a properly ordered, 'controlled', trial was not possible in conditions of disorder, and could have assisted his defence, in the presence of government and armed services representatives, of the MRC's failure to mount such a trial. In an apparently similar use of the term, the service representatives promptly agreed that 'it would be difficult to utilise service personnel in large groups for the controlled experiment for administrative reasons, leave, postings etc.' They did, however, suggest that they could provide 'small controlled groups probably of the order of 2,000'[92] for trials. 'Controlled groups' here appears to refer specifically to regulated, ordered populations. Some populations were, nevertheless, sufficiently stable for the MRC to contemplate a trial, enabling 'the possibility of controlled trials in camps of displaced persons'[93] or mental hospitals. Similarly, Stuart-Harris noted that, during his 1945/46 trial, 'the original arrangement to use vaccine in a controlled manner had broken down for reasons connected with the end of the war.'[94]

Describing the results of the winter 1946/47 trial in the *Lancet*,[95] Andrewes, Mellanby, Dudgeon and MacKay wrote that 'Prophylactic vaccination was carried out under controlled conditions during November and December, 1946....' The term 'controlled conditions' is not defined, but is at least partially a reference to stable populations; their report went on to describe the mental hospitals, public schools, preparatory schools, hospitals, Army training camps, prisoner-of-war camps, and other communities which they employed. But again, the rhetorical connotations of the term are apparent. 'Controlled conditions' conveys no additional description or information to the sentence within which it resides, but rather seems intended to persuade the reader of the ordered, efficient manner in which the study was conducted.

'Controlled' as 'efficient'

The remaining occurrences of the term 'controlled' appear to be intended to convey the impression of a properly ordered and planned, and efficiently executed, study. For example, the term was used to endorse the properly conducted status of British trials which had failed to demonstrate the impressive positive results achieved by the Americans. Stuart-Harris referred, in a lecture published in the *BMJ* in 1945, to studies in 1940 by Horsfall and Brown in the US which had demonstrated a protective effect of flu vaccine. The British trial on the same vaccine in 1941 had proved inconclusive, and Stuart-Harris felt it appropriate to single out this trial for description as 'controlled' – the only one so described in his entire lecture.[96] Similarly, the *BMJ* editorialist who applauded the positive results of the 1952 MRC study, attributed the inconclusive results of previous British trials to inadequate knowledge of antigenic variation in virus strains and to inadequate 'control' of field trials – apparently referring primarily to selection of comparison subjects. The 1952 trial had succeeded, however, because it was 'carefully controlled'.[97] Faced with a flu epidemic on the continent during the winter of 1948/49, the MRC planned a quick, small-scale trial 'in order to see whether anything could be achieved quickly, before an epidemic developed over here.' Nevertheless, lest this should imply inadequate planning, the trial was to be 'controlled'.[98]

This use of the term 'controlled' as 'rigorous' or 'efficient' also implies adequate standardisation of the vaccines under test. This concept is not unprecedented – drug standardisation was important to the MRC; for example, Cox has explored how the MRC defined and regulated the standardisation of insulin in the 1920s.[99] The discovery in 1940 that the vaccine supplied by the US contained live virus prompted the 'emphatic' decision not to use it unless it could be inactivated and could then pass British sterility tests – in which case Whittingham would consider its use in 'controlled inoculation experiments in the Air Force'.[100] Here 'controlled' apparently implies an imposition of order and efficiency by the British over the disorder induced by the American error. The MRC again used its 'controlled trials' to justify its requirements for superior quality vaccine in 1951 when its influenza vaccine committee agreed that 'controlled trials necessitate the preparation of stocks of vaccines which should be concentrated and purified and of a composition shown not to give rise to a significant incidence of reactions.'[101]

Conclusion

The use of comparison subjects – frequently referred to as 'controls' – was uncontroversial in trials of flu vaccine by this time, and the circumstances under which workers chose to describe their work as 'controlled' appear to owe far more to the rhetorical impact implicit in the use of the term, rather than simply to establish the presence of a comparison group. The term was used to justify MRC regulation of scarce vaccine supply and its refusal to allow stocks to pass to outsiders who requested them. It was used to emphasise the need for stable conditions in which to organise a proper trial, and hence to explain the MRC's failure to mount trials which could replicate the impressive American findings. Finally, it was used to endorse the proper design and conduct of British trials which nevertheless showed inconclusive results, and to justify the MRC's right to specify adequate vaccine quality.

By the time of the Second World War, the term 'controlled' had become embedded in MRC workers' notions of their work, of their right to arbitrate over the therapeutic efficacy of flu vaccine, and their right to determine its distribution. Their exploitation of the powerful rhetorical functions of the term are revealing. While the technical meaning of 'controlled' was hardening into a reference to comparison subjects, its other connotations were simultaneously becoming incorporated into MRC workers' concepts of the proper way to conduct their work. A controlled trial, with all that the term implies, was one which was played according to the MRC's tune.

Notes

1. Internet: http://www.uboat.net/allies/merchants/search.php [accessed 4 July 2007].
2. W.I.B. Beveridge, *Influenza: The Last Great Plague* (London: Heinemann, 1977), 24–6.
3. *Ibid.*, 27–30.
4. H.J. Parish, *Victory with Vaccines: The Story of Immunization* (Edinburgh: E. & S. Livingstone, 1968), 87; C. Langford, 'The Age Pattern of Mortality in the 1918-19 Influenza Pandemic: An Attempted Explanation Based on Data for England and Wales', *Medical History,* 46 (2002), 1–20.
5. Beveridge, *op. cit.* (note 2), 31.
6. Langford, *op. cit.* (note 4).
7. 'Minutes: Prevention of Influenza', 22 May 1951, FD1/540.
8. Beveridge, *op. cit.* (note 2), 2.
9. A. Chase, *Magic Shots: A Human and Scientific Account of the Long and Continuing Struggle to Eradicate Infectious Diseases by Vaccination* (New York: Morrow, 1982), 340.

10. *Ibid.*, 341–2.
11. Obituary, 'Wilson Smith', *British Medical Journal,* ii (1965), 240.
12. Obituary, 'Sir Patrick Laidlaw', *British Medical Journal,* i (1940), 551–2.
13. Obituary, 'Sir Christopher Andrewes', *British Medical Journal,* 298 (1989), 180.
14. Chase, *op. cit.* (note 9), 342.
15. Beveridge, *op. cit.* (note 2), 7–8.
16. W. Smith, C. Andrewes and P. Laidlaw, 'A Virus Obtained from Influenza Patients', *Lancet,* 2 (1933), 66–8.
17. Beveridge, *op. cit.* (note 2), 7–8.
18. Obituary, 'Charles Stuart-Harris', *British Medical Journal,* 314 (1997), 906–7.
19. Parish, *op. cit.* (note 4), 161.
20. Andrewes to Thomson, 14 October 1937, FD1/1113.
21. C.H. Stuart-Harris, W. Smith and C.H. Andrewes, 'The Influenza Epidemic of January–March, 1939', *British Medical Journal,* i (1940), 205–11.
22. Andrewes, Smith and Stuart-Harris, 'Memo', July 1939, FD1/1116.
23. Richardson to Mellanby, 20 July 1939, FD1/1116.
24. Laidlaw to Mellanby, 23 August 1939, FD1/1116. Serological testing for influenza virus involved inoculating ferrets and subsequently sacrificing them for post-mortem analysis.
25. Laidlaw to Mellanby, 23 February 1940, FD1/1116.
26. Andrewes, 'Memo', 24 June 1940, FD1/1116. Smith had first managed to cultivate the flu virus in chick embryos in 1935 – Beveridge, *op. cit.* (note 2), 9 – and Frank Macfarlane Burnet in Australia had developed a method to cultivate it in quantity by 1940, Parish, *op. cit.* (note 4), 162.
27. Andrewes , 'Memo', 19 July 1940, FD1/1116.
28. Parish, *op. cit.* (note 4), 162.
29. 'Notes on the Conference on Influenza Vaccine from the USA', 5 December 1940, FD1/1116.
30. Andrewes, 'Notes for Meeting', 9 July 1941, FD1/1116.
31. Andrewes, 'Notes for Meeting', 9 July 1941, FD1/1116.
32. Andrewes, 'Notes for meeting', 9 July 1941, FD1/1116.
33. Dale to Mellanby, 31 May 1941, FD1/1116.
34. Dale to Mellanby, 31 May 1941, FD1/1116.
35. Mackie to Mellanby, 19 August 1941, FD1/1116.
36. Mellanby to Andrewes, 20 August 1941, FD1/1116.
37. C.H. Stuart-Harris, 'Influenza Epidemics and the Influenza Viruses', *British Medical Journal,* i (1945), 251–7, 255.
38. Thomson to Sutherland, 12 November 1943, FD1/1116.
39. US Influenza Commission, 'The US Influenza Commission', *Journal of the American Medical Association* 124 (1944), 982.

40. 'Memo', [?] June 1944; undated and unsigned though the handwriting appears to be Andrewes', FD1/538.
41. 'Minutes: Vaccination Against Influenza', 30 June 1944, FD1/538.
42. 'Minutes: Vaccination Against Influenza', 30 June 1944, FD1/538, 3.
43. van den Ende, 'Memo', 24 August 1944, FD1/538.
44. Obituary, 'Sir Harold Whittingham', *British Medical Journal*, 287 (1983), 369.
45. 'Minutes: Vaccination Against Influenza', 29 November 1944, FD1/538.
46. Sirett to Herrald, 19 February 1945, FD1/538.
47. 'Minutes: Influenza Vaccination Conference', 29 June 1945, FD1/538.
48. Andrewes to Mellanby, 30 November 1945, FD1/538.
49. 'Draft Minutes: Conference on Influenza', 30 November 1945, FD1/538.
50. Stuart-Harris, 'Report: Trial of Influenza Vaccine', 15 July 1946, FD1/539.
51. Stuart-Harris, 'Report: Trial of Influenza Vaccine', 15 July 1946, FD1/539, 2. Also J.A. Dudgeon *et al.*, 'Influenza B in 1945-46', *Lancet*, 2 (1946), 627–31; Editorial, 'Influenza B', *Lancet*, 2 (1946), 644.
52. Stuart-Harris, 'Report: Trial of Influenza Vaccine', 15 July 1946, FD1/539.
53. 'Minutes: Conference on Influenza', 29 July 1946, FD1/539.
54. H. Mellanby et al, 'Vaccination Against Influenza A', *Lancet,* 1 (1948), 978–82.
55. 'Minutes: Influenza Vaccine', 21 January 1949, FD1/539.
56. 'Minutes: Prevention of Influenza', 1 October 1951, FD1/540.
57. 'Minutes: Prevention of Influenza', 22 May 1951, FD1/540.
58. J.C. Appleby, F. Himmelweit and C.H. Stuart-Harris, 'Immunisation with Influenza Virus A Vaccines: Comparison of Intradermal and Subcutaneous Routes', *Lancet*, 1 (1951), 1384–7.
59. Medical Research Council, 'Clinical Trials of Influenza Vaccine', *British Medical Journal,* ii (1953), 1173–7.
60. Himsworth, 'Memo', 20 November 1952, FD1/540.
61. McDonald to Wilson, 27 November 1952, FD1/540.
62. McDonald and Andrews, 'Preliminary Report on the Influenza Vaccine Trial in Luton, Winter 1952–53', FD1/540.
63. McDonald and Andrews, 'Preliminary Report on the Influenza Vaccine Trial in Luton, Winter 1952–53', FD1/540.
64. E.D. Kilbourne, 'A Race with Evolution: A History of Influenza Vaccines', in A.P. Plotkin and B. Fantini (eds.), *Vaccinia, Vaccination, Vaccinology: Jenner, Pasteur and their Successors* (Paris: Elsevier, 1996), 183–8.
65. 'Report: Trial of Influenza Vaccine', 15 July 1946, FD1/539, 1.
66. Editorial, 'The Prevention of Influenza', *British Medical Journal,* ii (1953), 1206–7.
67. See Wilson to Andrewes, 7 December 1945, FD1/538; Andrewes to Mellanby, 11 December 1945, FD1/538.

68. See 'Minutes: Vaccination Against Influenza', 29 November 1945, FD1/538, 3.

69. 'Influenza Vaccine Trials: Draft of Note to be Sent to the *British Medical Journal* and the *Lancet* with a Request for Publication in Issue of Week Ending November 29th', October 1952, FD1/540.

70. 'Statement for Press on Influenza Vaccine Trials', October 1952, FD1/540.

71. J. Liebenau, 'The MRC and the Pharmaceutical Industry: The Model of Insulin', in J. Austoker and L. Bryder (eds), *Historical Perspectives on the role of the MRC* (Oxford: Oxford University Press, 1989), 163–80.

72. D.C.T Cox-Maksimov, *The Making of the Clinical Trial in Britain, 1910–1945: Expertise, The State and the Public* (PhD thesis: Cambridge University, 1998), see Chapter 4, 'Biological Standards, Patients and the "Noble Scientists" of the MRC in the Insulin Trials: A Public Event', 131–77.

73. Liebenau, *op. cit.* (note 71), 169.

74. A.Y. Yoshioka, *Streptomycin, 1946: British Central Administration of Supplies of a New Drug of American Origin with Special Reference to Clinical Trials in Tuberculosis* (PhD thesis: Imperial College, University of London, 1998), see particularly Chapter 6.

75. B. Toth, *Clinical Trials in British Medicine 1858–1948, with special reference to the Development of the Randomised Controlled Trial* (PhD thesis: University of Bristol, 1998), see Chapter 5.

76. Yoshioka, *op. cit.* (note 74), 14.

77. Wilson to Andrewes, 7 December 1945, FD1/538.

78. Extract from Hansard, 8 November 1945, in FD1/538.

79. Wilson to Andrewes, 7 December 1945, FD1/538.

80. Andrewes to Wilson, 10 December 1945, FD1/538.

81. Wilson to Knox, 21 September 1946, FD1/539.

82. Wilson to Robinson, 6 December 1945, FD1/538.

83. 'Minutes: Prevention of Influenza', 22 May 1951, FD1/540.

84. 'Minutes: Vaccination Against Influenza', 29 November 1944, FD1/538, 3.

85. 'Minutes: Conference on Influenza Vaccine', 29 June 1945, FD1/538, 2.

86. Wilson to Andrewes, 7 December 1945, FD1/538.

87. Andrewes to Mellanby, 11 December 1945, FD1/538.

88. 'Minutes: Conference on Influenza', 30 November 1945, FD1/538, 3.

89. Richardson to Mellanby, 20 July 1939, FD1/1116.

90. 'Minutes: Conference on Influenza Vaccine', 29 June 1945, FD1/538.

91. 'Minutes: Conference on Influenza', 30 November 1945, FD1/538, 1.

92. 'Minutes: Conference on Influenza', 30 November 1945, FD1/538, 1.

93. 'Minutes: Conference on Influenza', 30 November 1945, FD1/538, 2.

94. 'Memo: Trial of Influenza Vaccine', 15 July 1946, FD1/539.

95. Mellanby, *op. cit.* (note 54).

96. Stuart-Harris, *op. cit.* (note 37), 255.
97. Editorial, *op. cit.* (note 66).
98. 'Minutes: Influenza Vaccine', 21 January 1949, FD1/539.
99. Cox-Maksimov, *op. cit.* (note 72), ch. 4.
100. 'Notes on the Conference on Influenza Vaccine from the USA', 5 December 1940, FD1/1116, 2.
101. 'Memo: Prevention of Influenza', 22 May 1951, FD1/540, 2.

Whose Words are they Anyway?
The Contrasting Strategies of Almroth Wright
and Bradford Hill to Capture
the Nomenclature of Controlled Trials

When Almroth Wright (1861–1947) began to endure the experience common to many new fathers, of sleepless nights caused by his crying infant, he characteristically applied his physiological knowledge to the problem in a deductive fashion. Reasoning that the child's distress was the result of milk clotting in its stomach, he added citric acid to the baby's bottle to prevent the formation of clots. The intervention appeared to succeed; Wright published his conclusions,[1] and citrated milk was eventually advocated by many paediatricians in the management of crying babies.[2]

By contrast, Austin Bradford Hill (1897–1991) approached his wife's insomnia in an empirical, inductive manner. He proposed persuading his wife to take hot milk before retiring, on randomly determined nights, and recording her subsequent sleeping patterns. Fortunately for domestic harmony, he described this experiment merely as an example – actually to perform it would, he considered, be 'exceedingly rash'.[3]

These anecdotes serve to illustrate the very different approaches to therapeutic experiment maintained by the two men. Hill has widely been credited as the main progenitor of the modern randomised controlled trial (RCT).[4] He was principally responsible for the design of the first two published British RCTs, to assess the efficacy of streptomycin in tuberculosis[5] and the effectiveness of whooping cough vaccine[6] and, in particular, was responsible for the introduction of randomisation into their design.[7] Almroth Wright remained, throughout his life, an implacable opponent of this 'statistical method', preferring what he perceived as the greater certainty of a 'crucial experiment' performed in the laboratory. In this chapter I shall examine the rhetorical strategies employed by Wright and Hill. The principal aim of this chapter is to emphasise the fundamental importance of rhetoric to workers in the emerging scientific discipline of therapeutic trial methodology. Unlike my analyses elsewhere, this does not focus uniquely upon the term 'controlled' but is a wider examination of the means by which the two protagonists attempted to capture the vocabulary, and hence the fundamental understanding, of the recently-described

Figure 6.1

Almroth Wright (1861–1947).
Courtesy: Wellcome Library, London.

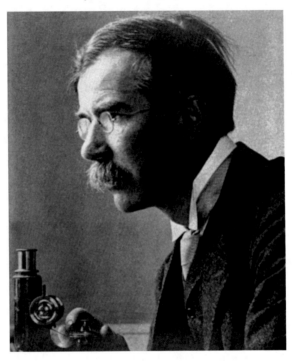

statistical therapeutic trial. The importance of this is far more than semantic; defining the words used to describe trial methodology allowed the protagonists to define, very differently, the very nature of therapeutic trials, the assumptions along which they must proceed, and the uses to which they may be put. This serves to emphasise the extraordinary potential, offered to workers involved in creating a discipline, of defining the nomenclature of that discipline; and particularly potent is Bradford Hill's adoption of the powerful term 'controlled'.

Wright invented a number of new words to supplement what he regarded as the deficient vocabulary of statistical experimentation. Bradford Hill, by contrast, adopted common words and phrases to describe new concepts. Wright's new words, and Hill's co-opted old ones, were ostensibly intended merely to provide precise terms for concepts where none had previously existed. Closer inspection reveals, however, that in naming these

Figure 6.2

Austin Bradford Hill (1897–1991)
Courtesy: Wellcome Library, London.

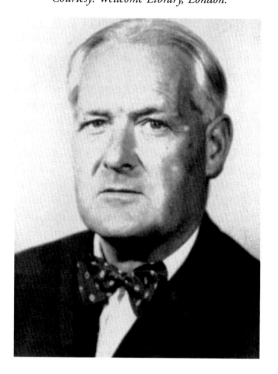

concepts Wright and Hill each subtly redefined them. An RCT designed and conducted using Wright's nomenclature would have been a far more constrained and circumscribed affair, with a far narrower range of uses, than one employing Hill's vocabulary. This analysis is intended to demonstrate the central importance of capturing the nomenclature of the RCT as a strategy to dictate the appropriate applications for such a trial and to dictate the people properly qualified to perform it. Wright described his ideas and nomenclature between 1912 and 1944, the early part of which occurs prior to Hill's work, but Wright's notions appear to have changed little over these three decades and although the two did not openly debate the virtues of statistical experimentation, their statements can be directly compared and contrasted.

Statistics in therapeutic experimentation

Recent authors have traced increasingly early origins for manipulation of numbers in British medicine, implying a quantification project spanning some three centuries. Seventeenth-century British quantifiers such as Francis Bacon and John Graunt – who analysed bills of mortality – inspired the eighteenth-century project of 'medical arithmetic' involving systematic quantification of population morbidity and mortality.[8] Regarding therapeutic experimentation, Ulrich Tröhler argues for the British origins of a quantitative, empirical approach to therapeutics from the beginning of the eighteenth century, arising in a community of like-minded, dissenting physicians who favoured meticulously recorded clinical observations and numerical quantification of case outcomes as the means to establish the most effective remedy.[9] Rosser Matthews traces the origins of 'statistics' in their current meaning – mathematical techniques to allow comparison of data – in British therapeutic experimentation to the biometrical tradition associated with figures such as Francis Galton and Karl Pearson during the last third of the nineteenth century.[10] This movement transformed statistics from the straightforward numerical description of social phenomena, into a mathematical discipline with techniques for analysing aggregated data. With the zoologist W.E.R. Weldon, Pearson and Galton founded the journal *Biometrika* in 1901, hoping to increase awareness of the value of mathematical statistics amongst the wider scientific community. Pearson, as Professor of Mathematics at University College London (UCL), ran a course on statistical theory, the only source for such instruction up to the 1920s. However, Matthews points out that throughout the 1920s and 1930s scientists in general, and medical practitioners in particular, remained sceptical of the application of statistical methods to their work.

Edward Higgs[11] has examined the incorporation of statistical methods into medical research through the establishment and efforts of the MRC Statistical Unit. He emphasises the importance of patronage relationships, exploited in particular by Major Greenwood (1880–1949), the first Director of the Statistical Unit. Greenwood and another key figure, George Udny Yule (1871–1951) had both received their statistics training from Pearson. Yule became Assistant Professor of Statistics at UCL in 1896 and a statistics lecturer at Cambridge in 1912, where he remained until his death in 1951. Greenwood undertook statistical work for the Ministry of Munitions during the First World War, where he met Walter Fletcher, the Medical Research Committee Secretary. The two developed mutual respect and a strong friendship, prompting Fletcher to persuade the Ministry to second Greenwood to the MRC in 1920, to chair the newly created Statistics Committee. The MRC's Statistical Unit, formed in 1914, had not performed well under what Fletcher perceived to be lacklustre direction by John Brownlee, and gradually became sidelined by the increasing activity of Greenwood's committee. Brownlee's death in 1928 enabled Fletcher to amalgamate the Statistical Committee and Statistical Unit as a single new MRC Statistical Unit under the leadership of Greenwood, who was by then Professor of Epidemiology and Vital Statistics at the London School of Hygiene and Tropical Medicine (LSHTM).

Greenwood was succeeded in the chair at LSHTM, and as head of the MRC Statistical Unit, by Bradford Hill in 1945. The web of patronage appears to have extended deeper even than Higgs has described. Greenwood had enjoyed considerable support in his own career from Hill's father, to whom he felt a debt of gratitude, which he repaid through his own patronage of Bradford Hill. Reflecting towards the end of his life, Bradford Hill considered that the help he received from Greenwood arose 'out of gratitude to and affection for my father.'[12] Indeed, he received sufficient patronage from Greenwood to conclude that, to him, 'I owed my whole career'.[13] Greenwood suggested that Hill study economics during his protracted convalescence (see below) and invited him to join him at the Statistical Committee in 1923, and again at LSHTM in 1933.

However, the extent to which the Statistical Unit and Committee influenced the methodology of therapeutic assessment in the MRC prior to the Second World War, is debatable. Higgs considers that from the mid-1920s, the MRC 'could proceed with applying the innovations of Pearsonian statistics to medical research'[14] and credits Greenwood and his subordinates with a wide and varied range of statistical examinations. Greenwood later reflected that the Statistical Committee 'had a large part in bringing statistical methods to bear upon laboratory researches as well as upon those field or rectory inquiries which admittedly involved statistical analysis.'[15] Writing in 1954, the then MRC secretary Francis Henry Knethell Green recalled that the MRC's Therapeutic Trials Committee (TTC), which existed from 1931 to 1939, had realised early in its life that 'the medical statistician is a valuable member of the planning team.'[16] Austoker and Bryder assert that 'expert opinion was frequently sought from the MRC's Statistical Committee' by the TTC,[17] a claim repeated by Matthews,[18] although neither attributes this claim and it might simply be a repeat of Green's statement.

However, the designs of the therapeutic trials conducted by the MRC prior to the 1940s appear to have been influenced very little by statistical considerations. When statisticians were approached the consultation appears to have occurred rather late in the day – Bradford Hill was responsible for the devastating *post-hoc* critique of the serum therapy trials, described in my chapter on serum therapy, and reflecting in 1986 on his involvement with the MRC during the 1920s and 1930s he considered that he and

Greenwood had 'worked hard and well in *correcting and improving* the statistics in the reports the Council proposed to publish,'[19] implying little involvement at the planning stage. Even for clinicians working on flu vaccine trials in the 1940s, statistical examination of their work was a *post-hoc* experience which generally amounted to a 'cold water douche,'[20] and Greenwood's published output prior to the 1940s appears to reveal more interest in epidemiology[21] and statistical experiments on mouse populations[22] than in any application of statistical methodology to therapeutic innovation. Iain Chalmers[23] has analysed the impact of statistical theory on Bradford Hill's thinking and upon the development of the RCT, and considers that formal statistical theory, for example, Ronald Fisher's writing on randomisation – had very little impact. Rather, he argues, Bradford Hill adopted randomisation in order to prevent doctors gaining foreknowledge of whether their patients were to receive active treatment. He points out that randomisation, often by alternation, had been an established technique since the early-twentieth century, and was adopted by workers such as Dora Colebrook in her light therapy study – described in my chapter on the MRC's trials of light therapy – without any reference to statistical theory, simply as a device to avoid subjective bias on the part of the investigators. Ben Toth[24] similarly presents the MRC's adoption of statistics into trial design largely as a rhetorical device to enhance the apparent scientific objectivity of their work, rather than as an enterprise driven by any underlying statistical theory. Cox[25] claims that her analysis of the MRC files reveals no evidence of written consultation between statisticians and clinicians during this period. She concludes that not until the TTC was disbanded at the onset of the Second World War did the MRC begin to reconfigure the therapeutic trial as a mechanised mass event devised by statisticians such as Hill.[26] Nor did Hill appear to claim that trials prior to the mid-1940s were much influenced by statistical theory; he regarded the first of his RCTs to be published, the streptomycin trial,[27] as a very different affair to anything which had gone before. He certainly regarded this trial as having a novel design at the time.[28] As discussed in the introductory chapter of this work, it constituted 'a landmark in medical research',[29] and formed a model for future work, albeit with subsequent refinements.[30]

The empiricist: Austin Bradford Hill

Austin Bradford Hill was born in 1897 to a prestigious family; his great-great uncle, Sir Rowland Hill, had introduced the penny post and his father was an eminent professor of physiology at the London Hospital.[31] A keen sportsman in his youth, Hill delayed his entry to medical school in order to serve as a pilot during the First World War. The devastating blow to his health came, not from flying – he emerged unscathed from his only crash, at the Chingford reservoirs – but on the Greek islands in 1917, when he contracted near-fatal pulmonary tuberculosis and was invalided home to die. After nine months in bed, and a therapeutically induced pneumothorax, he eventually began to recover, although two years' convalescence meant that his days as a sportsman, and his aspirations to study for a medical degree, were at an end. He gleefully pointed out, towards the end of his life, that he subsequently received his hunded per cent disability pension for over seventy years.

At Greenwood's suggestion, Hill used his convalescence to enrol in an external degree in economics at the University of London in 1918, studying through his own reading and a 'rather ineffectual' correspondence course.[32] After gaining his economics degree in 1922 he attended, and was inspired by,[33] part of Pearson's statistics course at UCL. Medicine remained his primary interest, however, and he avidly read textbooks both of medicine and statistics.[34] Meanwhile, his patron Greenwood, who was instrumental in arranging an MRC grant to allow Hill to study mortality in country districts, brought him onto the MRC Statistical Committee in 1923, and again to a readership in epidemiology and vital statistics at the LSHTM in 1933. During the Second World War, Hill was seconded to the Research and Experimental Department of the Ministry of Home Security, but became disillusioned when his carefully researched report demonstrating that Anderson air-raid shelters were effective, was promptly 'marked secret and locked in a drawer'[35] – whereupon he moved to the Medical Directorate of the Royal Air Force.

In 1945 Hill succeeded Greenwood in his chair at LSHTM and as head of the MRC Statistical Unit, remaining in both positions until his retirement in 1961. He also held positions as a member of the MRC, consultant to the Royal Navy, member of the Committee on the Safety of Medicines, Secretary of the Royal Statistical Society, and from 1950 to 1952 as President of the Royal Society. He was knighted in 1961.

Hill considered the RCT to be a new tool, requiring a new set of ethical considerations.[36] The factors that he considered new about these trials were:

[T]he most careful *planning* of the experiment in advance, and an experiment that usually, though not invariably, makes the following demands: (a) the construction of two (or more) closely similar *groups* of patients observed at the same time and differing in their treatment; (b) the construction of these groups by some process of *random* allocation; and (c) the *withholding* of a form of treatment from one or other of these groups.[37]

These factors – statistical planning, and a randomised, controlled design – chiefly characterise the trials which Hill was ultimately to refer to simply as 'controlled clinical trials'. Others also used terms such as 'controlled trials,' 'statistical-clinical trials', 'statistical trials', or 'statistical experiments'. These terms appear to have been used interchangeably throughout the 1930s, 1940s and 1950s and I shall assume in the following analysis that they were, in this context, synonymous.[38]

Hill was to become fervent in his claims that a properly conducted trial must involve statistical considerations from the very start, meaning not only that the statistician should be 'in it up to his neck... that is, at the initial planning level,'[39] but also that the clinicians involved must themselves be conversant with basic statistical theory and technique; he argued that the resulting collaboration between statisticians and clinicians should ideally prove synergistic.[40] His first opportunity to persuade clinicians to the advantages of statistics came shortly after his appointment to the LSHTM, when he was given responsibility for teaching statistics to medical postgraduates.[41] The potential opportunity to influence an entire generation of clinicians arose when he published these lectures in 1937 as a series of seventeen weekly articles in the *Lancet,* and then as a textbook, *Principles of Medical Statistics.*[42] The book remained in print for twelve editions until 1991, and was translated into numerous languages. In its pages, Hill outlined statistical theory and the design of a 'controlled trial', rendering him, as Cox[43] has pointed out, the first statistician publicly to claim clinical trials as his territory. Hill enhanced the considerable[44] influence of *Principles of Medical Statistics* by lectures and articles over the following three decades, and chaired an international conference in Vienna in 1959, at which the controlled trial was presented as a uniquely British model for therapeutic research.[45]

The rationalist: Almroth Edward Wright

Almroth Wright, one of medicine's 'most picturesque characters',[46] was born in Yorkshire to a Swedish mother and an Irish father – a fiery clergyman given to loud and angry denunciation of Rome.[47] Wright spent his childhood in Dresden and Boulogne, where his father held livings, then spent fifteen years studying in Ireland. His father's clerical income did not permit Wright to indulge his academic whims and he largely paid for his own education by winning scholarships. He emerged with a degree in literature and subsequently one in medicine, from Trinity College Dublin, and took a Grocers' travelling scholarship to study physiology in Germany. Returning to England, he found that medical practice did not appeal and so returned to study – this time the law, with a view to a position at the Bar. This, too, was unappealing once his studies were completed whereupon Wright accepted a clerkship in the Admiralty.[48]

Finally settling upon a career in laboratory medicine, Wright took demonstratorships in pathology at Cambridge in 1887, then two years later in physiology at Sydney. He returned to England to take the professorship of pathology at the Army Medical School at Netley in 1891, where his work on blood coagulation provided the basis for his attempts to quieten his sleepless infant with citrated milk.[49] He travelled to India to serve on the Plague Commission in 1898, testing his recently-developed typhoid vaccine, and on his return was appointed pathologist at St Mary's Hospital in London in 1902, where he remained for the rest of his career. Much of his work was concerned with developing and promoting 'vaccine therapy' – the employment of immunisation in the treatment of established infective disease, rather than simply as a prophylactic measure. By 1910 vaccine therapy was in its heyday, universally praised as 'a triumph for English medicine and for Sir Almroth Wright',[50] and Wright as its main progenitor was lauded as 'epoch making.... The British Pasteur'.[51] Although vaccine therapy was subsequently largely abandoned, Worboys considers it of fundamental importance in enhancing the prominence and importance of laboratory medicine in Britain prior to the First World War.[52]

Wright's colleague Leonard Colebrook recorded that human suffering disturbed Wright – he never got used to walking though wards full of wounded and sick men in order to reach his laboratory during the First World War[53] – and that much of his laboratory work was aimed at producing direct therapeutic benefit. He worked on wound sepsis and gas-gangrene during the First World War, during which time his department at St Mary's produced four and a half million doses of anti-typhoid vaccine – a mass inoculation programme which was credited with saving the lives of around 125,000 servicemen.[54] He was knighted in 1906.

An 'uncompromising individualist'[55] Wright expected nothing less than the fullest commitment from his staff, whom he regularly kept out of their beds into the early hours, several nights a week[56] – although midnight usually brought a break for a cup of strong tea and a discussion of one of Wright's favoured topics, most notably the shortcomings of the female intellect.[57] His friend George Bernard Shaw characterised him in *The Doctors' Dilemma* as the scientific, if pedantic, Sir Colenso Ridgeon.[58] The portrayal apparently did not meet with Wright's wholehearted approval, for upon seeing the play for the first time he left in disgust during the interval.[59] Wright was nevertheless a tireless advocate of the primacy of the laboratory as the proper place to generate scientific, medical, and therapeutic knowledge.[60] He maintained that many physiological and therapeutic experiments were simply impossible to perform *in vivo*, and that only the laboratory offered the regulation of variables essential for a 'crucial experiment',[61] claiming, 'The all-important thing in science is not measurement but *certainty*.'[62] He reserved his most scathing criticism, however, for 'statistical experimentation' and the limited men of 'mediocre ability'[63] whom he perceived to be its practitioners.

Almroth Wright and the validation of therapeutic efficacy

Wright's opinion of the statistical method was first born out of a series of clashes with statisticians, principally Greenwood and Pearson, which have been documented by Matthews.[64] Wright, in 1904, published a treatise claiming success for his anti-typhoid inoculation, which Pearson countered with a highly critical statistical analysis. The two clashed further over the reliability of the opsonic index, a measure devised in 1902 by Wright and his colleague at St Mary's, Captain Stewart Douglas. Wright postulated a substance in blood serum, opsonin, which facilitated the ingestion of bacteria by leucocytes. Measuring the activity of opsonin in a serum sample could, he claimed, provide a reliable laboratory measure of antibacterial activity and even detect infection while the patient was still asymptomatic, and would revolutionise medical therapy. Wright considered that measurement of the opsonic index should also guide the dosage of vaccine therapy for an individual patient. The opsonic index appears, however, to have been little used outside Wright's laboratory, and although vaccine therapy enjoyed considerable popularity during the first decade of the twentieth century it appears that most practitioners employed it without resort to the opsonic index.[65] Greenwood's criticisms, on mathematical grounds, of the opsonic index helped cement his early career as a statistician; at the heart of the ensuing debate was Greenwood and Pearson's conviction that biometrics and statistical analysis offered a means to obtain scientific knowledge. Wright rejected the notion of a role for a professional mathematical statistician, in favour of laboratory immunology and bacteriology.[66]

Wright regarded the laboratory as the primary place to generate therapeutic certainty, with clinical therapeutic experimentation having largely a secondary, confirmatory role. His proposed treatment for war wounds, for example, was derived entirely from laboratory findings and physiological principles.[67] This confidence in laboratory validation appeared to survive even in the face of bitter personal experience. Whilst at Netley, Wright developed a vaccine against Malta fever; once his laboratory experiments had demonstrated that the vaccine successfully induced antibodies against the causative organism, *Brucella melitensis*, Wright expected that it would therefore prove therapeutically effective. He inoculated himself with the vaccine, then ingested live *B. melitensis* organisms. It was several months before he fully recovered from the devastating bout of Malta fever that followed.[68] Wright's convictions regarding the value of laboratory experimentation in determining therapeutic efficacy nevertheless remained unshaken. A single, properly-conducted, 'crucial' laboratory experiment would suffice: 'One experiment suffices, if properly performed, to establish the truth of a principle.... To devise a crucial experiment is a work of genius.'[69]

Even when the time came to assess the effect of a new therapy upon a human subject, Wright was dismissive of clinical acumen, preferring the certainty of laboratory measurement to assess a patient's condition – one of his favourite tricks to make his point, was to hide a half-crown coin under some blankets and challenge clinicians to use their allegedly sharply-honed palpation skills to find it.[70] He was equally sceptical of clinicians' abilities to judge whether a treatment was of genuine value; discussing the therapeutics of bacterial infection, he reasoned that patients treated with topical antiseptics frequently improved following therapy, but also frequently deteriorated. 'Clinical observation,' he concluded, 'leaves us in incertitude as to whether a method of treatment is doing a modicum of good, or a modicum of harm, or is doing neither good nor harm.'[71] Rather, it was necessary to invoke the laboratory as an arbiter of therapeutic efficacy: 'We must, in order to discover the event of a therapeutic intervention, have recourse to laboratory technique and scientific apparatus.'[72]

Nevertheless, Wright accepted that once a drug had proven its worth in the laboratory then some form of clinical testing was necessary, in what he described as a real world outside the laboratory where repeatable phenomena could not be relied upon and one had to tolerate a degree of uncertainty. In this uncertain world, Wright concluded that 'there will needs have to come into application a new logic and a new technique of reasoning.'[73] He described two possible approaches – the 'experiential' method, in which clinicians use the impressions that they have accumulated after repeated experiences with the new drug to arise at generalisations, and the statistical method.[74] The statistical method he regarded as limited, as it could only address a single outcome, and observations by different practitioners could not easily be pooled and directly compared. The experiential method he regarded as better aligned with the process by which humans naturally form impressions and accumulate knowledge. The judicious and experienced clinician would scrutinise *all* the features of each case, not simply those which had been selected in advance as outcome measures. With repeated observations of different cases, anomalies would stand out and so would easily be discounted, and the observer's mind would filter out any factors of importance.[75] Wright quoted a number of complicated case histories in which the success or failure of vaccine therapy was not readily apparent; the statistical method would be 'hopeless' in investigating such cases, he asserted, appealing instead to the judgement of the judicious, impartial, clinical observer to unpick the complexities of such case histories in the uncertain world outside the laboratory.[76]

Quoting a number of examples where he regarded this experiential method to have proven its value – the use of sulphur ointment to treat itching, quinine for malaria, salvarsan in syphilis, and staphylococcal or streptococcal vaccines for local infections[77] – Wright proposed as an important clinical arbiter of therapeutic efficacy, the establishment through the experiential method of a medical consensus, 'The fact that the medical profession, so far as it has experience of these remedies, is *unanimous* in its favourable verdict is evidence that they are signally effective.'[78] This view appeared to find some favour with his clinical colleagues; at a discussion on vaccine therapy at the Royal Society of Medicine in 1910 the existence of a consensus in favour of the treatment was taken as proof of its 'self-evident' efficacy,[79] and the opinion expressed that 'the difficulty in estimating the value of a new remedy is greatly exaggerated.'[80] Wright,[81] and his followers such as Alexander Fleming,[82] frequently quoted isolated case reports as evidence of the clinical utility of remedies which they regarded as having already proved themselves in the laboratory, apparently regarding such case reports as a form of crucial clinical experiment which lent support to existing laboratory findings; large-scale clinical trials had little or no place in this hierarchy of evidence. The laboratory, then, ruled supreme; the necessary clinical testing of remedies could frequently be performed on a small scale, and experienced clinicians should find little difficulty in reaching a consensus regarding a treatment's worth through careful clinical observation.

Guided by these principles, Wright deemed the statistical method wholly inappropriate when the time came for clinical trials of a new drug, ethyl hydrocuprein hydrochloride ('optochin'), which had shown promising laboratory activity against *Streptococcus pneumoniae* in Germany. Rather, he administered the drug to just eight Africans who had contracted pneumonia, and relied upon his own judicious clinical observation combined with laboratory measurement of the subjects' opsonic index to ascertain its effects. Optochin proved to have a devastating side-effect; two patients were permanently blinded, apparently by the treatment, which in any case appeared to be 'dubiously effective'.[83] Although distressed at this outcome, Wright nevertheless regarded it as a vindication of his methodology which had identified the drug's toxic effects and dubious efficacy with a fraction of the number of patients – and of cases of blindness – that a statistical trial would have demanded.[84]

Wright did, however, allow some place for the statistical trial in the evaluation of large-scale prophylactic measures,[85] or circumstances where there was little discernible difference between treated and control subjects,[86] and performed a number of large-scale trials of inoculation against pneumonia upon 'natives' in Africa. He first satisfied himself of the activity of his pneumococcal vaccine by demonstrating a rise in the opsonic index of subjects who were inoculated with it in his laboratory. He administered the vaccine therapeutically to 159 patients admitted to the Witwatersrand Native Labour Association Hospital in Johannesburg and compared its effects against 149 untreated controls, allocated by alternation. The intervention appeared to be 'absolutely ineffective'[87] – fifty treated subjects died, compared with forty-eight untreated – although Wright remained convinced by his laboratory findings that the vaccine did work, explaining away his results with reference to incorrect dosing and the low resistance of African natives in comparison to white subjects.[88]

A larger study of prophylactic inoculation followed, subjects again being randomised to receive inoculation or no treatment by alternation. The vaccine appeared to exert an effect; sixty-one deaths occurred amongst 5,963 subjects inoculated, compared with 116 deaths in the 5,671 'controls'.[89] Wright then attempted a more ambitious, larger-scale study of prophylactic inoculation in 20,000 to 30,000 Africans, again with alternate allocation to treatment or 'control.' Despite Wright's best efforts to instruct his medical and administrative staff in the correct procedures for the investigation, a degree of organisational chaos ensued, and the study had to be abandoned.[90] Many subjects were lost to follow-up, the study population turned out to be composed of a number of different tribal and racial groups, and there were differences between controls and treated subjects particularly with regard to race. Significantly, Wright appeared to regard these problems, not as flaws in the design and execution of his study, but as defects inherent to the very nature of a large-scale statistical trial. His earlier trial, in India, of typhoid vaccine during 1898 and 1899 involved 11,295 subjects and had also proved something of a shambles; Wright was not able to administer all the doses of vaccine himself and was reliant on local medical officers for treatment and follow-up of subjects, tasks which they performed with highly variable degrees of diligence.[91] Record-keeping was frequently shoddy and sometimes even deliberately faked.[92] Wright subsequently regarded the fact that a statistical trial required large numbers of subjects and therefore a substantial number of investigators some of whom would be 'inferior medical practitioners',[93] as a further reason why such trials were generally impractical.

There followed, in May 1912, a 'new experiment on better lines'[94] investigating a more limited sample of 8,800 Africans; a further two similar trials ensued. Wright concluded from these six trials that his pneumonia vaccine was effective. He performed no statistical analysis upon the results, which he appeared to regard as self-evident.[95] Even then, one of his most significant conclusions arose from deduction and the use of laboratory data to extrapolate from his results, rather than from the mortality figures he presented. Wright noted that the small number of subjects who were unfortunate enough co-incidentally to develop pneumonia within six days of having received their prophylactic immunisation, appeared to enjoy a lower death rate than similarly unfortunately infected 'controls' – though characteristically, he provided no statistical analysis to support this claim. Wright argued that this implied a therapeutic effect of the vaccine when administered in the early stages of pneumonia. He argued from his laboratory-acquired knowledge:

> [A]s we know that the bacterioclastic power of the blood does not sensibly increase, when pneumonia develops, we think it reasonable to suppose that the favourable results which were obtained... would repeat themselves if this treatment were applied in the early stages of pneumonia.[96]

Although Wright did not openly debate the merits of the statistical trial with Bradford Hill, he continued to articulate and publish his views throughout the 1930s and 1940s, up to his death in 1947. During this time Hill was developing and promoting his ideas on clinical trials, and devising the methodology for the MRC's streptomycin and whooping cough trials. The following analysis examines contemporaneous pronouncements of the two men concerning therapeutic experimentation and contrasts their rhetorical strategies, in order to demonstrate that language and nomenclature were of pivotal importance in forming notions of what should properly comprise therapeutic experimentation.

The right word for the job

Exposition and correct vocabulary, were of paramount importance to Wright. As part of what George Bernard Shaw described as 'his efforts to excogitate a scientific method of reasoning,'[97] Wright invented a considerable number of new words – many of which appear to be a rendition of a relatively mundane English term into Latin.[98] Even a partial listing of these neologisms occupies three pages in Wright's biography by his colleague and erstwhile disciple, Sir Zachary Cope.[99] Wright regarded new words as an intrinsic part of any genuine scientific advance: 'Words are the custodians of ideas (Mill). Each advance is signalized by the invention of a new word.'[100] Shaw considered that these were 'new and necessary words'[101] for fields whose vocabulary had hitherto been deficient; the leader writer in the *Lancet*, on the occasion of Wright's death, appeared less convinced, noting faintly that of Wright's many neologisms, possibly 'some... will survive'.[102]

Wright was not alone in placing a high value on linguistic precision in the making of scientific knowledge. The notion was central to much philosophical thought during the first half of the twentieth century; the philosophy of logical positivism arose during the 1920s among philosophers and scientists of the 'Vienna Circle' and was influential in Britain throughout the 1930s.[103] Central to its doctrine was the notion that philosophical questions are largely questions of language. A crucial question within logical positivism, related to where meaning resides within a statement. A logical positivist would only consider a statement meaningful if it could be verified – either empirically, or through rigorous logic. The meaning of a statement therefore resided within its method of verification, and the primary focus of the philosophy was directed towards language and meaning, rather than knowledge.[104] Linguistic precision was of fundamental importance to this style of analysis. The British philosopher, Bertrand Russell, subsequently worked to develop a hierarchy of language, arguing that a statement in one language could only be considered valid in relation to another, higher-level language. Ultimately, he argued, it should be possible to infer real properties of the world from a properly-constructed, logically purified form of language.[105]

Wright's views on language were broadly shared by a number of workers in emergent fields of medicine such as laboratory scientists and specialists, who were largely responsible for provoking a contrary resurgence of 'neo-Hippocratism' in inter-war Britain.[106] Neo-Hippocratists tended to ally with the 'patrician' physicians described in my first chapter, who reacted against the systematisation, professionalism, and reductionism in medicine which they saw as contingent upon the increasing influence of laboratory science, specialists, and state interference. Words were important in the debate; naming something, claimed the neo-Hippocratists, imbued it with a spurious reality. Labelling a disease, for example, created a false, simplified entity which did not reflect the complex reality of diagnosis – which, they argued, required experience and tacit knowledge rather than simply application of textbook learning. The neo-Hippocratists were scornful of those who were taken in by words as representations of abstract concepts, considering these individuals limited in imagination and ideas; they particularly criticised those such as Wright who constructed neologisms from imported Greek terms.

Wright, however, considered a correct and precise vocabulary to be essential for the advance of any endeavour and that its absence implied an immature discipline peopled by workers of limited ability. He regarded the vocabulary of the statistical trial to be particularly lacking and considered that this reflected very poorly upon its practitioners. Any field of learning which was well stocked with terminology represented, he reflected, 'a study which has attracted to its service generations of men of pre-eminent ability.'[107] By contrast, 'a terminology which fails to provide words for quite fundamental notions…' represented 'a science which has attracted to its service only men of mediocre ability.'[108] The statistical trial was such a science: 'The vocabulary of *Statistical Experimentation* is... distressingly defective.'[109] Frequently, he considered, its terminology included words for specific cases but not the generic; for example, there existed no generic term for those receiving a therapeutic intervention in a controlled trial, but only specific terms – 'the treated', 'the inoculated', 'the dieted'. Wright employed this example to put the practitioners of statistical experimentation in their proper intellectual place alongside primitive tribesmen, 'a terminology which supplies *specific* but no *generic names* – has distinctly barbaric affinities.'[110] He likened statisticians to the aborigines of Tasmania, who had a name for each species of tree but no generic word for 'tree', or the Zulus who had a word to distinguish each variety of cow but no generic term for 'cow'.

Wright set about correcting these perceived deficiencies in the vocabulary of statistical experimentation. He proposed that subjects receiving intervention should be termed 'inscripts', and those not receiving the intervention be termed controls or 'contra-scripts'. He distinguished 'se-ispic' or 'auto-proteric' controls, where the condition of a patient before treatment is compared with the condition of the same patient after treatment, and 'allotrious isochronous' controls where a group of inscripts is compared with a group of contra-scripts.[111] Inscripts and contra-scripts must, he maintained, be similar in all important respects, and must be subjected to identical conditions including their risk of infection.[112]

The intervention being tested by the trial, Wright termed the 'erg'. However, he also used this term to refer to any other physical agent which could affect the trial's outcome; multiple ergs could act simultaneously and it was therefore important to ensure that 'no physical "*Erg*", other than the one we propose to investigate, shall intrude into our experiment.'[113] Besides ergs, a trial could also be confounded by 'advects' – 'any passive agent which might, by quenching or buffering, nullify the action of the erg whose action we are investigating.'[114] Wright referred to the set of people under investigation as the 'community', and explained that he preferred this term to the statistician's 'population'.[115] The measurement which was to be used to determine the outcome of the trial, Wright designated the 'eventus',[116] and stressed that the eventus must be chosen so as to admit only an unequivocal 'yes' or 'no' response to whatever question the trial was posing.

Even where existing statistical vocabulary did provide its own terms, Wright was dismissive. He criticised statisticians' use of the term 'significant' – although whether through deliberate disengenuity, or through ignorance of contemporary statistical concepts, he chose to define the term very differently to the statisticians. Wright identified a statistically significant result as one involving a difference of at least ten per cent in magnitude between 'inscripts' and 'contra-scripts' at the completion of a trial.[117]

Statisticians at the time employed instead a probabilistic definition of significance, an outcome with a less than one-in-twenty probability of having occurred by chance being regarded as significant.[118] Wright's definition of the term 'probable error' was similarly non-mathematical,[119] and he also criticised the statistical term 'random sampling', largely on the grounds that it was tautologous – any sampling worthy of the name should, he maintained, be random.[120]

Wright offered his neologisms in order to fill the 'notable *lacunae* in the vocabulary of statistical experimentation.'[121] However, his terminology potentially achieved far more than that. The words he provided were not simply direct replacements for existing statistical notions; in naming these concepts Wright re-defined them. The overall effect was to change and substantially diminish the role of any statistically controlled trial conceived and executed employing his terminology. Wright was opposed to the widespread use of statistical trial methodology and his new nomenclature served subtly to constrain and diminish its application. In order to develop this theme, let us contrast Wright's approach with the rhetorical style of Bradford Hill.

Plain and simple; statistics for the uninitiated

In contrast to Wright, Bradford Hill preferred to adapt existing words to serve in his vocabulary of statistics, generally choosing terms which would already be familiar to his non-mathematical audience. Contemporaries commended his writing and speaking styles for their clarity and avoidance of mathematical terminology or statistical jargon.[122] On the rare occasion that he did feel constrained to introduce a new term, he did so almost apologetically – when, with Richard Doll, he coined the adjective 'prospective' to describe a trial which follows its participants into the future, he carefully provided a definition from the Oxford English Dictionary to support his new use of the term.[123] He explained the specific meanings of words which he did adopt, for example elaborating upon 'the meaning which the statistician attaches to the word "selected"'[124] in his discussion of sample selection. In his *Principles of Medical Statistics* he frequently expressed mathematical formulae as text rather than mathematical symbols, for example rendering the formula for calculation of Chi-squared as:

$$(\text{Observed number} - \text{expected number})^2 \,/\, \text{Expected number}[125]$$

Hill shared none of Wright's difficulty with the absence of a generic term for those receiving intervention in a controlled trial, for example referring variously to 'the inoculated',[126] 'the immunised',[127] or the 'treated'.[128] The trial's outcome measures he referred to as 'the criterion of success or failure'[129] and in later publications also as 'the questions asked of the trial',[130] simply

157

'measurements,'[131] or even 'adding up the score at the end of play',[132] in contrast to Wright's neologistic 'eventus'. This use of common terminology and avoidance of specialist or mathematical terms was, Hill later claimed, quite deliberate; reflecting on his 1937 *Principles of Medical Statistics*, he stated in 1990:

> I deliberately left out the words 'randomization' and 'random sampling numbers' at that time, because I was trying to persuade the doctors to come into controlled trials in the very simplest form and I might have scared them off... I thought it would be better to get doctors to walk first, before I tried to get them to run.[133]

These sentiments also illustrate Hill's notions of the nature of his audience. He was writing and speaking for practising clinicians, who had little grounding – and frequently, little interest – in statistics or mathematical theory. Even the medical postgraduates whom he taught at the LSHTM 'had little liking or aptitude for mathematics',[134] and clinicians in the wider world were frequently even less receptive.[135] His chosen vehicle for publication was the *Lancet*, until he quarrelled with its editor and shifted his allegiance to the *BMJ*[136] – both journals were accessible to the mainstream of practising clinicians. His strategy of coercing mathematically reluctant medics by straightforward words and phrases was one which he was later to regard as having been successful; in 1952 he considered that, although it was a bold step for a statistician to venture into areas 'in which are practised the arts of the clinician', it was nevertheless a step which he had by then 'been fortunate enough to be able to take.'[137] Hill regarded the conversion of the mainstream medical profession to statistical methodology as his primary aim, and as one of his finest achievements; receiving his honorary MD at Edinburgh from Professor John Croft in 1968, he cautioned: 'You know I did not invent the controlled trial. It goes back at least to Lind.' 'I know that', replied Croft, 'But you persuaded an extremely conservative profession which regarded change with suspicion, to accept and use them.' Hill later reflected, 'That was, and is, I think, a fair judgement.'[138]

Wright's intended audience, by contrast, appears to have been simply those clinicians and scientists who were amenable to his views. Rather than attempt to cajole the medical mainstream, he denounced roundly those clinicians untrained in laboratories.[139] He published almost entirely in the mainstream medical journals – *Lancet, BMJ* and *Proceedings of the Royal Society*[140] – but his uncompromising approach hardly appeared calculated to persuade the medical masses; Henry Dale reflected that:

> [H]is findings and his presentation of them were apt to excite opposition and dispute – partly, no doubt, because he himself so enjoyed the clash of

opinion and the cut and thrust of argument, with a well-grounded confidence in his own prowess.[141]

Grab the vocabulary, and their hearts will follow

The terminology being developed for the statistical trial, was of fundamental importance in forming notions of the trial amongst the medical community. Providing a nomenclature for a scientific discipline offers a degree of control over the very nature of that discipline and of the concepts it is possible to maintain within it. This is far from a novel insight, as briefly discussed in my introductory chapter. Jan Golinski, for example, describes how Lavoisier's new chemical nomenclature constrained thinking to within the boundaries of his own system of chemistry, a criticism which was indeed levelled at the time.[142] Lavoisier's own defence to these charges appears reminiscent of Wright's statements, by claiming that a precise and accurate nomenclature is essential to the progress of any new science: 'if languages are really instruments fashioned by men to make thinking easier, they should be of the best kind; and to strive to perfect them is indeed to work for the advancement of science....'[143] Dudley Shapere emphasises the importance of naming and defining concepts before a new scientific discipline can address them; for example, he maintains that it would be impossible to have a debate about the process of star formation until the term 'star' had acquired a certain, specific meaning.[144]

Compare an imaginary controlled trial employing Wright's nomenclature with one using Hill's terminology, and we have two very different affairs. The intervention under test is, according to Hill 'the treatment'; usually it is quite rigidly defined, although this need not be the case,[145] and Hill subsequently allowed clinicians where necessary to vary dose regimes according to individual patients' idiosyncrasies.[146] Wright's 'erg' allows no such variation; each erg in every experiment must be qualitatively and quantitatively the same.[147] Furthermore, in Wright's scheme the erg under investigation is merely one of a number of ergs acting simultaneously. Together with the action of numerous 'advects', these potentially represent myriad confounding factors, which render difficult or impossible the task of separating the action of the erg under investigation. Designing our trial under Wright's nomenclature therefore becomes a more complex affair, involving the difficult task of identifying and nullifying this multiplicity of confounding factors, compared to Hill's nomenclature which enables us to concentrate upon the single 'treatment' and even to vary it as necessary to suit the needs of our patient. Hill's response to potentially confounding factors – Wright's 'ergs' and 'advects' – was largely to nullify them through random allocation of treated and control subjects; as discussed below, this notion is also implicit in Hill's terminology.

Wright drew his subjects from a 'community' of persons, objecting to the statisticians' term 'population'.[148] Although he did not explain the reasons for this preference, the term 'community' implies a collection of individuals with rights and responsibilities who are interacting, mutually dependent, and whose actions will affect others; according to the *Oxford English Dictionary (OED)*, 'social intercourse, fellowship, communion... life in association with others, society.'[149] A 'population', on the other hand, could be taken to represent simply an aggregation of people without implicit interaction, as in the *OED*'s definition: 'the total number of persons inhabiting a country, town, or other area.'[150] A mutually interacting 'community' thus implies a less favourable environment than a 'population' in which to isolate the effect of a chosen erg, since any attentions of others in the community could confound or confuse the effects of the erg under study. Simply by adopting Wright's preferred term here, our study is beset with potential difficulties which are not implicit in Hill's terminology. A further problem when we are designing our trial according to Wright's nomenclature is that his 'community' must be composed of persons who are all 'fundamentally similar', particularly with regard to age and race.[151]

Hill's terminology offered fewer implicit obstacles; he drew ultimately from a 'universe' of people, meaning *all* people theoretically amenable to study – for example, in a study on treatment for diabetes, the 'universe' would be all the diabetics in the world.[152] From this 'universe' a 'population' was selected, comprising the subjects who were to be involved in the study.[153] These terms do not carry the same implications of complex social interaction as Wright's term 'community'. Nor was it essential for Hill's 'population' to consist of 'fundamentally similar' individuals, as was the case with Wright's 'community'. Although this happy state would be desirable, Hill maintained that it was still possible to study a more diverse population by applying statistical techniques such as stratification or frequency distribution,[154] and by random allocation of control or treated subjects.[155] The constraints upon our imaginary trial in terms of the range of conditions and subjects who we can study, appear far fewer when the trial is planned using Hill's vocabulary.

Having identified the 'community' or 'population' to be studied, the next step in our imaginary trial is to choose the participants. If we are adopting Wright's nomenclature and searching for 'inscripts' and 'contra-scripts' then we must look for individuals whom Wright defined as 'in every important respect, similar.'[156] This represents an extremely difficult task, because of individual variation – Wright cautioned that 'even patients who are suffering from one and the same infection cannot, because of the great differences which prevail among them, be equitably assorted... into comparable groups of *'Inscripts'* and *'Contra-scripts.'* [157] He then went on to ridicule the notion that alternation could achieve 'any equitable assortment of patients'. Hill, by contrast, proposed random allocation as a solution to the problem of equitable selection – initially by strict alternation,[158] and by the time of his streptomycin and whooping cough trials, by random numbers – 'because *in the long run* we can fairly rely upon this random allotment of the patients to equalise in the two groups the distribution of other characteristics that may be important.'[159] Wright's 'inscripts' and 'contra-scripts' are not, therefore, the same as Hill's 'treated' and 'control' subjects, but are more narrowly defined, and more difficult and laborious to identify. A trial employing them would be a more limited affair than one designed under Hill's terminology, and in some circumstances would not even be possible at all.

Once our imaginary study is completed, we must analyse the results. Under Wright's terminology, we should inspect the 'eventus'. Since Wright was concerned that 'one can very seldom feel complete confidence in purely clinical results,'[160] his 'eventus' must be entirely objective, and chosen 'as to admit of the question asked being answered in terms of an unqualified "yes" or an unqualified "no".'[161] This stipulation considerably limits the scope of our trial, as few clinical outcome measures are quite so unequivocal, with the exception of death, which, fortunately, rarely constitutes a suitable end-point for a trial.[162] Employing Hill's terminology, we look simply to 'measurements', which should be as objective as possible, but which can also incorporate subjective clinical assessment. Hill dismissed attempts to adopt overly-objective criteria as rather missing the wood for the trees:

> [W]e must never overlook – as has been emphasized this week – that objective bits and pieces may not present a coherent picture of the whole. If the sedimentation rate falls, the pulse is steady and the blood pressure impeccable, we are still not very much better off if unfortunately the patient dies. The clinical judgement of the whole is, or may be, still fundamental.[163]

Once again, Wright's 'eventus' imposes constraints on the scope of our trial which are not implicit in Hill's 'measurements'.

The consequence of adopting Hill's terminology in designing a controlled trial is therefore to enable an enterprise far broader in scope, capable of asking and answering a far wider range of questions, than is possible under the narrower constraints imposed by Wright's nomenclature. Although the terminology developed by the two men ostensibly defined the same concepts, the subtleties of definition were sufficient to render two very different notions of a therapeutic trial. Wright, employing his new nomenclature to reinforce his argument, concluded that 'isochronous, allotriously controlled, statistical experimentation, is (as we have seen) inapplicable to the testing of remedial agents.'[164] Hill, by contrast, looked forward to his version of the controlled trial being increasingly employed in the future to evaluate the burgeoning numbers of new drugs and other treatments, such as physiotherapy.[165]

A controlled trial or a statistical trial?

The foregoing analysis is intended to demonstrate the importance of semantics in establishing the role, scope, and very nature of the emerging statistical trial. By defining differently the statistical trial's terms, Wright and Hill each presented a very different picture of the trial to the medical establishment. Historically, Hill's terminology, and hence his notions of a properly constituted statistical trial, have dominated. Wright's neologisms are now obsolete, and none will be found in a modern textbook. The contrast between the two systems nevertheless demonstrates the extent to which common notions of the statistical trial have been formed by its terminology – in other words, by Hill's terminology. Employing, wherever possible, words familiar to a non-mathematical medical readership, Hill promoted a trial which was inclusive – not only inclusive of all doctors in its intended audience, but inclusive of a far wider range of patients and problems for study than Wright's limited affair.

Hill also exploited the rhetorical connotations of a 'controlled' trial. He utilised the term increasingly as his notions of trial methodology developed, until – by the time of the 1948 streptomycin trial – a 'controlled clinical trial' had become Hill's and the MRC's shorthand for a properly conducted trial. Alternative descriptions such as 'statistical trial' faded from the scene during the 1950s, and by 1959, Hill and his MRC colleagues could convene an international conference entitled simply 'controlled clinical trials' to present what they regarded as a particularly British model for therapeutic research.[166] Hill and his colleagues consolidated the term 'controlled clinical trials' throughout the 1950s, but an analysis of this process is outside the scope of this work; however, a brief analysis of the increasing use which Hill made of the term 'controlled' up to the publication of the 1948 streptomycin trial should help establish that by this time, he had effectively adopted the term, and its rhetorical connotations, to describe *his* version of a therapeutic trial.

In early editions of his *Principles of Medical Statistics,* Hill used the term 'controlled' only once, apparently to indicate the presence of appropriately selected comparison subjects. In the context of a discussion of the allocation of patients into control and treatment groups, he concluded: 'In the long run it is probable that useless forms of treatment will be discarded and the good will survive, but it may be an unfortunately long run which carefully controlled trials would have effectively shortened.'[167] He employed other terms besides 'controlled trial' to identify his methodology, including 'clinical trial'[168] and – in an echo of Wright's preferred term 'statistical trial' – 'the statistical method'.[169]

With the fourth edition of *Principles of Medical Statistics* in 1948, the same year as the publication of the streptomycin study, Hill staked his claim to the term 'controlled trial' as a shorthand description of his methodology. Although much of the book remained largely unchanged, a new section noted that: 'In the first and last chapters of this book emphasis is laid upon the necessity for controlled trials of a new form of treatment....'[170] The first and last chapters were unaltered from previous editions and made no specific mention of 'controlled trials' other than the one reference noted above. However, Hill now chose to characterise the methodology to which these chapters referred, as 'controlled trials'. In doing so, he was adopting a term which was already in common use by MRC workers to describe their own studies – which, as described elsewhere in this work, had hitherto represented a diverse and idiosyncratic collection of methodologies. Inevitably, along with the term, Hill borrowed its rhetorical associations, which he successfully applied exclusively to his RCT methodology.

Notes

1. A.E. Wright, 'On the Possible Advantages of Employing Decalcified Milk in the Feeding of Infants and Invalids', *Lancet*, ii (1893), 194.

2. Editorial, 'Sir Almroth Wright', *British Medical Journal*, i (1947), 646–7.

3. A.B. Hill, 'Medical Ethics and Controlled Trials', *British Medical Journal*, i (1963), 1043–9, 1045.

4. See for example, R. Doll, 'Austin Bradford Hill', *Biographical Memoirs of Fellows of the Royal Society*, 40 (1994), 129–40; J.R. Matthews, *Quantification and the Quest for Medical Certainty* (Princeton: Princeton University Press, 1995), Chs 6 and 7.

5. Medical Research Council Streptomycin in Tuberculosis Trials Committee, 'Streptomycin Treatment for Pulmonary Tuberculosis', *British Medical Journal*, ii (1948), 769–82.

6. Medical Research Council, 'The Prevention of Whooping-Cough by Vaccination', *British Medical Journal*, i (1951), 1463–71.

7. R. Doll, 'Austin Bradford Hill', *Lancet*, 337 (1991), 1154; see also Chapter 1 of this volume.

8. See for example, G. Jorland, A. Opinel, and G. Weisz (eds), *Body Counts: Medical Quantification in Historical and Sociological Perspective* (Montreal: McGill-Queen's University Press); for a related analysis concerning the nineteenth-century origins of statistical thinking in the United States, see J.H. Cassedy, *American Medicine and Statistical Thinking, 1800–1860*. (Cambridge: Harvard University Press, 1984).

9. U. Tröhler, *"To Improve the Evidence of Medicine:" The Eighteenth Century British Origins of a Critical Approach* (Edinburgh: Royal College of Physicians of Edinburgh, 2000); U. Tröhler, 'Quantifying Experience and Beating Biases: A New Culture in Eighteenth-Century British Clinical Medicine', in Jorland, *op. cit.* (note 8), 19–50.

10. Matthews, *op. cit.* (note 4), Ch. 5.

11. E. Higgs, 'Medical Statistics, Patronage and the State: The Development of the MRC Statistical Unit, 1911–1948', *Medical History,* 44 (2000), 323–40.

12. A.B. Hill, *The Start and Early Years of my Career* (Manuscript collection of the London School of Hygiene and Tropical Medicine, 1988).

13. *Ibid.*

14. Higgs, *op. cit.* (note 11), 336.

15. M. Greenwood, 'The Statistician and Medical Research', *British Medical Journal,* ii (1948), 467–8: 467.

16. F.H.K. Green, 'The Clinical Evaluation of Remedies', *Lancet,* ii (1954), 1085–90.

17. J. Austoker and L. Bryder, 'The National Institute for Medical Research and Related Activities of the MRC', in J. Austoker and L. Bryder (eds.), *Historical Perspectives on the Role of the MRC* (Oxford: Oxford University Press, 1989), 35–57: 46.

18. Matthews, *op. cit.* (note 4), 129.

19. A.B. Hill, 'Introduction', in M. Greenwood, *The Medical Dictator and other Biographical Studies* (London: Keynes Press, 1986), xi (my italics).

20. This comment is referenced in my chapter 5, concerning the MRC's flu vaccine trials.

21. For example, see E.L. Collis and M. Greenwood, *The Health of the Industrial Worker* (London: J. and A. Churchill, 1921).

22. For example, see M. Greenwood, *Experimental Epidemiology* (London: HMSO, 1936).

23. I. Chalmers, 'Statistical Theory was Not the Reason that Randomization was Used in the British Medical Research Council's Clinical Trial of Streptomycin for Pulmonary Tuberculosis', in G. Jorland, *op. cit.* (note 8), 309–34.

24. B. Toth, *Clinical Trials in British Medicine 1858–1948, with special reference to the Development of the Randomised Controlled Trial* (PhD thesis: University of Bristol, 1998).

25. D.C.T. Cox-Maksimov, *The Making of the Clinical Trial in Britain, 1910–1945: Expertise, The State and the Public* (PhD thesis: Cambridge University, 1998), 203.

26. *Ibid.,* 205.

27. Medical Research Council, *op. cit.* (note 5).

28. See the accompanying *BMJ* editorials to the streptomycin trial (Editorial,

'Streptomycin in Pulmonary Tuberculosis', *British Medical Journal,* ii (1948), 791–2; Editorial, 'The Controlled Therapeutic Trial', *British Medical Journal,* ii (1948), 791–2.) Although these were unattributed, Chalmers considers that Hill almost certainly wrote the streptomycin editorial – Chalmers, *op. cit.* (note 23) – which described the trial as 'the first of its kind'.

29. R. Doll, 'Sir Austin Bradford Hill and the Progress of Medical Science', *British Medical Journal,* 305 (1992), 1521–6.
30. *Ibid.*
31. *Ibid.*; Obituary, 'Sir Austin Bradford Hill', *British Medical Journal,* 302 (1991), 1017; Doll, *op. cit.* (note 7); Doll, *op. cit.* (note 4).
32. Doll, *op. cit.* (note 4), 130.
33. Hill in his unpublished memoirs credits Pearson's lectures, and Udny Yule's textbook *The Theory of Statistics,* with inspiring his interest in statistics. Hill, *op. cit.* (note 12).
34. *Ibid.*
35. *Ibid.*
36. Hill discussed the ethics of controlled trials in numerous published articles, but see particularly A.B. Hill, 'Aims and Ethics', in Council for International Organizations of Medical Sciences, *Controlled Clinical Trials: Papers Delivered at the Conference Convened by the Council for International Organizations of Medical Sciences* (Oxford: Blackwell, 1960), 3–7, and Hill, *op. cit.* (note 3).
37. Hill, *op. cit.* (note 3), 1044 (his italics).
38. For an example of various of these terms being used interchangeably see Editorial, 'Out, Damned Spot', *British Medical Journal,* ii (1951), 1074–5. 'Statistical trial' and 'statistical experiment' were terms particularly beloved of Almroth Wright, see below.
39. A.B. Hill, 'The Clinical Trial', *New England Journal of Medicine,* 247, 4 (1952), 113–19: 114.
40. Hill, 'Aims and Ethics', *op. cit.* (note 36), 7.
41. Doll, *op. cit.* (note 4), 131.
42. A.B. Hill, *Principles of Medical Statistics,* 1st edn (London: The Lancet, 1937).
43. Cox-Maksimov, *op. cit.* (note 25), 205.
44. See for example, Doll, *op. cit.* (note 4), 132, for an assessment of Hill's impact on clinicians.
45. A.B. Hill, 'Conclusion: The Statistician', in Council for International Organizations of Medical Sciences, *op. cit.* (note 36), 168–71.
46. Editorial, *op. cit.* (note 2).
47. L. Colebrook, 'Almroth Edward Wright', *Lancet,* i (1947), 654–6.
48. *Ibid.*
49. Obituary, 'Sir Almroth Wright', *British Medical Journal,* i (1947), 657–8.
50. W.D. Emery, 'Vaccine Therapy', in A.E. Wright, *Vaccine Therapy, its*

Administration, Value and Limitations (London: Longmans, Green & Co., 1910), 187–97: 190.

51. M. Worboys, 'Vaccine Therapy and Laboratory Medicine in Edwardian Britain', in J. Pickstone (ed.), *Medical Innovations in Historical Perspective* (Basingstoke: Macmillan, 1992), 84–103: 85.

52. *Ibid.*

53. Colebrook, *op. cit.* (note 47), 655.

54. Obituary, *op. cit.* (note 49).

55. Editorial, *op. cit.* (note 2).

56. D.W. Carmalt-Jones, 'Sir Almroth Wright', *Lancet,* i (1947), 930.

57. Colebrook, *op. cit.* (note 47), 655. Wright also published his anti-feminist views; A.E. Wright, *The Unexpurgated Case Against Woman's Suffrage* (London: Constable, 1913).

58. J. Freeman, 'Sir Almroth Wright', *British Medical Journal,* i (1947), 659–60.

59. M. Dunnill, *The Plato of Praed Street: The Life and Times of Almroth Wright* (London: Royal Society of Medicine Press, 2000), 240.

60. See for example, A.E. Wright, 'On Vaccine Therapy and Immunisation in Vitro', *Lancet,* ii (1931), 225–30, 225.

61. A.E. Wright, *Studies on Immunisation,* 2nd ser. (London: W. Heinemann, 1944), 237–40. Wright's 'crucial experiment' was one performed in a laboratory, with all variables regulated, such that repeating the same experiment under identical conditions would inevitably produce an identical outcome.

62. *Ibid.*, 247 (his italics).

63. *Ibid.*, 240.

64. Matthews, *op. cit.* (note 4), Ch. 5.

65. Worboys, *op. cit.* (note 51), 93.

66. Matthews, *op. cit.* (note 4), Ch. 5.

67. A.E. Wright, 'An Address on Wound Infections: And on some Methods for the Study of the Various Factors which come into Consideration in their Treatment', in A.E. Wright, *Pathology and Treatment of War Wounds* (London: Heinemann, 1942), 1–29.

68. Dunnill, *op. cit.* (note 59), 38. Dunnill, a pathologist, provides an explanation for the vaccine's failure in terms of twenty-first century pathology; the vaccine was ineffective because it induced humoral immunity, mediated through antibodies, whereas the immune response against B. melitensis is predominantly cell-mediated.

69. L. Colebrook, *Almroth Wright: Provocative Doctor and Thinker* (London: Heinemann, 1954), 240.

70. Dunnill, *op. cit.* (note 59), 40.

71. Wright, *op. cit.* (note 61), 225.

72. *Ibid.*, 225.

73. A.E. Wright, *On Pharmaco-Therapy and Preventive Inoculation applied to Pneumonia in the African Native* (London: Constable, 1914), 19.
74. *Ibid.,* 20.
75. *Ibid.,* 23.
76. A.E. Wright, *Vaccine Therapy, its Administration, Value and Limitations: A Discussion Opened by Sir Almroth E. Wright* (London: Longmans, Green & Co., 1910), 34–7.
77. Wright, *op. cit.* (note 73), 37.
78. *Ibid.,* 39 (his italics).
79. J.W. Eyre in Wright, *op. cit.* (note 76), 60–4: 61.
80. J.K. Fowler in Wright, *ibid.*
81. Wright, *ibid.*
82. A. Fleming in Wright, *ibid.,* 137–9.
83. Wright, *op. cit.* (note 73), 44–5.
84. Dunnill, *op. cit.* (note 59), 129.
85. Wright, *op. cit.* (note 61), 246.
86. Wright, *op. cit.* (note 73), 25.
87. *Ibid.,* 84.
88. Dunnill, *op. cit.* (note 59), 131.
89. Wright, *op. cit.* (note 73), 89.
90. *Ibid.,* 89.
91. Dunnill, *op. cit.* (note 59), 59–60.
92. Wright, *op. cit.* (note 61), 244.
93. *Ibid.,* 244.
94. Wright, *op. cit.* (note 73), 91.
95. *Ibid.,* 91.
96. *Ibid.,* 104.
97. G.B. Shaw, 'Sir Almroth Wright', *British Medical Journal,* i (1947), 659.
98. See, for example, Wright's section on 'Crucial experimentation', Wright, *op. cit.* (note 61), 237–40.
99. Z. Cope, *Almroth Wright: Founder of Modern Vaccine-Therapy* (London: Nelson, 1966), 116–18.
100. This is one of a collection of Wright's aphorisms recorded in Colebrook, *op. cit.* (note 69), 238.
101. Shaw, *op. cit.* (note 97).
102. Editorial, *op. cit.* (note 2).
103. O. Hanfling, 'Logical Positivism', in S.G. Shanker (ed.), *Routledge History of Philosophy, Vol. IX: Philosophy of Science, Logic and Mathematics in the 20th Century* (London: Routledge, 1996), 193–213.
104. *Ibid.,* 195.
105. F. Copleston, *A History of Philosophy: Vol. VIII, Bentham to Russell* (London: Search Press, 1966), 462–9.

106. The following account derives from D. Cantor, 'The Name and the Word: Neo-Hippocratism and Language in Interwar Britain', in D. Cantor (ed.), *Reinventing Hippocrates* (Aldershot: Ashgate Pub., 2002), 280–301.

107. Wright, *op. cit.* (note 61), 240.

108. *Ibid.,* 240.

109. *Ibid.,* 241.

110. *Ibid.,* 241 (his italics).

111. *Ibid.,* 241.

112. *Ibid.,* 243.

113. *Ibid,* 237–8.

114. *Ibid.,* 238

115. *Ibid.,* 242.

116. *Ibid.,* 243.

117. *Ibid.,* 242.

118. A.B. Hill, *Principles of Medical Statistics,* 2nd edn (London: The Lancet, 1939), 86, also 67, where Hill offers a mathematically near-equivalent probabilistic definition of significance as a difference greater than twice the standard error.

119. Wright, *op. cit.* (note 61), 242.

120. *Ibid.,* 242.

121. *Ibid.,* 241.

122. T. Fox, 'Foreword', in Hill, *op. cit.* (note 42), iii–iv; Doll, *op. cit.* (note 4), 131–2.

123. R. Doll and A.B. Hill, 'The Mortality of Doctors in Relation to their Smoking Habits', *British Medical Journal,* i (1954), 1451–5, 1451.

124. Hill, *op. cit.* (note 118), 9.

125. *Ibid.,* 82.

126. *Ibid.,* 94.

127. *Ibid.,* 128.

128. *Ibid.,* 177.

129. *Ibid.,* 176.

130. A.B. Hill, *Principles of Medical Statistics,* 6th edn (London: The Lancet, 1955), 238.

131. Hill, *op. cit.* (note 39), 117.

132. *Ibid.,* 117.

133. A.B. Hill, 'Memories of the British Streptomycin Trial in Tuberculosis', *Controlled Clinical Trials,* 11 (1990), 77–9: 77.

134. Doll, *op. cit.* (note 4), 131.

135. For examples of clinicians' scepticism towards the usefulness of mathematics and statistics in therapeutic research see for example, J.N. Badham, 'More Blasts on the Trumpet', *British Medical Journal,* ii (1951), 1218; T.O. Williams, 'More Blasts on the Trumpet', *British Medical Journal,* ii (1951),

1218; A.S. Barr, 'More Blasts on the Trumpet', *British Medical Journal,* ii (1951), 1218–49, and subsequent correspondence.

136. Hill, *op. cit.* (note 12).
137. Hill, *op. cit.* (note 39), 113.
138. Hill, *op. cit.* (note 12).
139. M. Greenwood, 'Almroth Edward Wright', *Lancet,* i (1947), 656.
140. L. Colebrook, *Bibliography of the Published Writings of Sir Almroth E. Wright, MD, FRS* (Toronto: Heinemann Medical Books, 1952).
141. H. Dale, 'Almroth Edward Wright', *British Medical Journal,* i (1947), 659.
142. J. Golinski, *Making Natural Knowledge: Constructivism and the History of Science* (Cambridge: Cambridge University Press, 1998).
143. Lavoisier in 1787, cited from L. Hogben, *The Vocabulary of Science* (London: Heinemann, 1969), 28.
144. D. Shapere, 'On Deciding what to Believe and how to Talk about Nature', in M. Pera and W. Shea (eds.), *Persuading Science: The Art of Scientific Rhetoric* (Canton: Science History Publications, 1991), 89–103.
145. Hill suggests that rigid definition of treatment is not necessary provided that the treatment remains consistent. A.B. Hill, *Principles of Medical Statistics,* 4th edn (London: The Lancet, 1948), 193–4.
146. Hill, *op. cit.* (note 39), 117.
147. Wright, *op. cit.* (note 61), 243.
148. *Ibid.,* 242.
149. *Oxford English Dictionary, Second Edition* (Oxford: Oxford University Press, 1989)
150. *Ibid.*
151. Wright, *op. cit.* (note 61), 243.
152. Hill, *op. cit.* (note 118), 9.
153. *Ibid.,* 11.
154. *Ibid.,* 20.
155. *Ibid.,* 5.
156. Wright, *op. cit.* (note 61), 243.
157. *Ibid.,* 245 (his italics).
158. Hill, *op. cit.* (note 118), 5.
159. *Ibid.,* 5 (his italics).
160. Wright, *op. cit.* (note 61), 244.
161. *Ibid.,* 243.
162. Hill, *op. cit.* (note 39), 117.
163. Hill, *op. cit.* (note 45), 169.
164. Wright, *op. cit.* (note 61), 249.
165. Hill, *op. cit.* (note 45), 168.
166. Hill, *op. cit.* (note 36).
167. Hill, *op. cit.* (note 118), 173; A.B. Hill, *Principles of Medical Statistics,* 3rd

edn (London: The Lancet, 1942), 173.

168. Hill, *op. cit.* (note 118), 172; Hill, *Principles,* 3rd edn, *op. cit.* (note 167), 172.

169. Hill, *op. cit.* (note 118), 172, 179; Hill, *Principles,* 3rd edn, *op. cit.* (note 167), 172, 179.

170. Hill, *op. cit.* (note 145), 193.

7

Conclusion:
What's Controlled about the Controlled Trial?

Should the gastroenterologist Harold Conn suffer the misfortune to bleed from oesophageal varices,[1] he would hope to be included in a randomised controlled trial, enter the trial, and then refuse treatment.[2] Thus he would maximise his chance of successful recovery – for simply being selected for a trial is a powerful predictor of a favourable outcome. Subjects entered into a radomised controlled trial (RCT) are likely to be carefully diagnosed, free from other serious diseases, and compliant with their treatment and any strictures it imposes. They will receive meticulous clinical scrutiny from doctors following a careful treatment protocol, and probably also from additional supplementary staff.[3] Thus, most RCTs are designed to assess what the British epidemiologist Archie Cochrane designated *efficacy* – whether a treatment can possibly work, under the idealised conditions of a trial – rather than what he called *effectiveness*, whether the treatment works in real-life clinical practice. A third question concerns the treatment's *efficiency*, or whether its benefits are worth the resources it consumes.[4]

This work has examined the utilisation, by physicians associated with the MRC, of the powerful rhetorical connotations of the term 'controlled' in order to promote their own work in therapeutic assessment prior to the publication of the MRC's streptomycin trial in 1948. These therapeutic trials were idiosyncratic affairs and the methodology of a proper clinical trial was, at this time, neither unified nor codified. But the MRC nevertheless referred consistently to its own trials as 'controlled'. The term encompassed an eclectic assortment of methodologies and carried a variety of rhetorical associations. The unifying characteristic which bound the various uses of the term 'controlled', was its use as a rhetorical device at a time when the authority to determine the proper means of testing a remedy was very much up for grabs. Ultimately, the MRC's 'controlled trial' became a construct – prior to 1948 there was no single methodology which could define the term, no published trial which could exemplify it, yet the 'controlled trial' was exploited as a rhetorical device to enhance the authority of a therapeutic experiment performed under the auspices of the MRC. However, the rhetorical associations of the 'controlled trial' did not disappear abruptly with the codifying of RCT methodology in 1948; they remain inherent to the discourse on therapeutic efficacy today – where debate still attends the RCT, and more broadly the field of evidence-based medicine (EBM), within which the RCT is embedded.

The randomised controlled trial after 1948

The MRC continued to promote its newly-defined controlled trial as the model for therapeutic evaluation and its members were heavily involved in an international conference in Vienna in 1959, staged to promote RCT methodology.[5] By 1966, Hedley Atkins, President of the Royal College of Surgeons of England, felt able proudly to proclaim 'the controlled clinical trial' as 'an almost exclusively English contribution to medicine.'[6] Scientific evidence now dictated therapeutic decision-making, he claimed:

> [T]he advocacy of a therapeutic measure depends now, not on the force of personality, the standing in the profession, or the 'mellifluidity' of the protagonist, but on more soundly based scientific evidence, and the tool for the forgoing of this evidence is the controlled clinical trial.[7]

Few present-day advocates of EBM would be likely to quibble with this as a succinct exposition of their philosophy.

The trickle of RCTs published in international medical journals expanded steadily throughout the 1950s and 1960s, multiplied dramatically in the 1970s and early-1980s, and reached a peak in the mid-1980s before apparently falling back to levels equivalent to the 1970s over the following decade.[8] This decline is probably artefactual, due to increased reporting of RCTs in the recently-burgeoning numbers of specialist journals which were not examined in these surveys; analysis of online databases suggests that actual RCT numbers continue to rise.[9] There appears to have been a trend to larger studies, involving more participants, over the past two decades.[10] At the same time, the number of published meta-analyses has increased substantially.[11] Meta-analysis is a statistical technique whereby the results of a number of RCTs which have all investigated the same therapeutic intervention, are aggregated and analysed en masse, thereby increasing the statistical power of the investigation. It can enable a definitive statistical conclusion to be drawn from disparate RCTs with differing sample sizes, and which might even reach differing individual conclusions; it occupies an important place at the top of the hierarchy of evidence employed by present-day EBM practitioners. Meta-analysis is distinct from systematic review, where reviewers attempt to locate all good-quality trials relating to a therapy and reach a conclusion based upon their assessment of the evidence provided by each individual trial, rather than by statistical analysis of aggregated results – although systematic reviewers might well consider meta-analyses alongside individual trials. Systematic reviews have formed a mainstay of the

EBM initiative, particularly in Britain where the influential Cochrane Library includes a database of systematic reviews, and their number has increased substantially over the past couple of decades.

A number of influential commentators have examined the factors underlying the rapid rise in the quantity of RCTs, and in the faith placed in them by the medical profession and the public, over the latter half of the twentieth century. Most narratives acknowledge the importance of the thalidomide tragedy. Thalidomide was promoted during the 1950s as a treatment for pregnancy sickness and was responsible for a global epidemic of infants born with deformed or stunted limbs – phocomelia. Although the infant population of the United States escaped almost unaffected due to delays in licensing the drug, the thalidomide debacle nevertheless expedited legislation mandating the American Food and Drug Administration to regulate the drug industry,[12] and prompted similar initiatives internationally. Proof of *efficacy* was for the first time considered intrinsic to establishing a drug's *safety*, placing the RCT centre stage in drug regulation.

Theodore Porter, in an influential volume, defines two types of objectivity within professional communities – 'disciplinary objectivity' and 'mechanical objectivity'. Disciplinary objectivity arises by consensus from experienced senior members of the community, who employ tacit knowledge – judgement that can only arise from experience and training. Mechanical objectivity is rule-based, frequently employing quantification and numbers, and does not depend on incommunicable wisdom and experience. When an expert community faces a perceived threat, argues Porter, it transfers its legitimacy from disciplinary to mechanical objectivity. Tacit knowledge and expert opinion might still carry some weight within the profession, but its public rhetoric emphasises science and the objectivity implied by numbers. So the Western medical establishment, under threat during the latter twentieth century in many countries from large, frequently state-controlled medical organisations, resorted to placing its trust in numbers and prioritised the controlled trial.[13] Harry Marks[14] prefers to consider the RCT in the United States as a device employed by academic physicians intent on therapeutic reform, who sought a tool to distinguish effective from ineffective remedies and curb the enthusiasm for excessive prescribing amongst their non-academic colleagues. By forging an alliance with statisticians these practitioners could acquire the tool they needed – the RCT – while giving the statisticians a boost to their hitherto meagre prestige in the medical hierarchy. In a related analysis, Jeanne Daly suggests that the rise in popularity of public health medicine during the 1950s and 1960s led to blurring of the boundaries between clinical medicine, social care. and politics. In danger of being consumed entirely by issues of social justice and poverty and becoming, effectively, social workers, physicians adopted the

RCT as a research tool which provided scientific credibility to public health work. By adopting only interventions established as effective by an RCT, physicians defined their role more narrowly and excluded murkier areas of activity.[15]

The RCT in the twenty-first century

Harold Conn, who we encountered at the beginning of this chapter, is not alone in his cynical view of the relevance of RCT findings to the wider world. The development and execution of RCTs is a multi-billion pound industry – unsurprising, given the current hegemonic position of the RCT as the gold standard for evaluating therapeutic efficacy. But critics of the RCT have by no means gone away over the past fifty years. Trial methodology has frequently been insufficiently rigorous in the past as a result of which, according to Sir Iain Chalmers – one of the developers of the British Cochrane Collaboration, whose database of controlled trials and systematic reviews has been most influential in promoting EBM worldwide – 'a massive amount of research effort, the goodwill of hundreds and thousands of patients, and millions of pounds have been wasted.'[16] Particular problems can attach to RCTs designed to assess, for example, surgical procedures,[17] complex social interventions,[18] or performed on children.[19] Patients are generally motivated to participate in trials through perceived self-benefit rather than altruism;[20] they frequently object to, or fail to understand, the notion of random allocation,[21] and are particularly apt to decline recruitment into a trial containing a placebo arm.[22] Authors including Evelleen Richards[23] and Steven Epstein[24] have described how patient resistance to aspects of methodology such as randomisation and placebos, led to protocol modification of RCTs investigating HIV therapy in the United States during the 1980s. Practitioners have even questioned the validity of comparing a therapy against placebo at all, arguing that this denies the importance of human factors and the doctor–patient relationship in healing.[25] Persuading physicians to recruit patients into a trial may also prove difficult, due to operational factors in a busy clinic, doctors' ethical concerns about randomisation, or their lack of faith in the intervention under test.[26] Even when an RCT does provide an unequivocal result, doctors frequently find it difficult to apply its population-based conclusions to the individual patient facing them.[27]

Modifications of RCT methodology have been proposed, and adopted, to address some of these concerns – patient preference trials, in which patients with a strong preference receive their chosen therapy, with others being randomised;[28] 'n-of-1' trials in which the effects of a drug are compared with placebo (or another drug) in a single patient;[29] cluster randomised trials, where whole sets of patients are randomised together;[30]

standardised complex intervention trials, where complex interventions are redefined and treated as simple ones;[31] 'computrials' where no comparison subjects are recruited, but controls are identified instead from existing computer records;[32] and even a return to non-randomised, observational trials.[33]

However there are other, more fundamental, gripes with the RCT. One is the concern that its dominance has channelled medical research into questions which can only be answered by an RCT, thereby sidelining issues which are important in practice such as the therapeutic power of the doctor–patient interaction, and the idiosyncratic requirements of individuals when it comes to making real treatment decisions.[34] Another problem is how to interpret and apply RCT results. The eminent epidemiologist Richard Peto and the MRC scientist Colin Baigent bemoan the fact that clinicians not infrequently draw the 'wrong conclusions' even from good-quality, large-scale RCTs and advise physicians how to approach trial results in order to avoid such errors.[35] But their caveats assume that there is a single 'right conclusion' to draw from the results of an RCT. Recent scholarship has examined the interpretation and application of RCT findings in social and political context and argues that such considerations are essential to understanding the use which has been made of RCT results. Evelleen Richards describes trials of vitamin C in the treatment of cancer during the 1970s and concludes that establishment physicians ultimately rejected the therapy, not through consensus over the results of trials, but because it represented a threat to their own conceptual authority. 'Evaluation,' she comments, 'may be better understood as inherently a political process,'[36] and she warns that the effectiveness of the RCT 'is increasingly compromised by patient and consumer resistance to its principle of randomization and by professional resistance to the implementation of those of its findings that conflict with established professional practices.'[37]

James McCormack and Trisha Greenhalgh have analysed the interpretation by authors, editors, and the wider scientific community of a large RCT, the United Kingdom Prospective Diabetes Study (UKPDS) which was published in 1998. They describe how commentators drew conclusions from the study which were not supported by the data, but which accorded with the commentators' own professional or political agendas. They conclude that: 'Biases arise when different stakeholders assign their individual values to the interpretation of the final results of randomised controlled trials.'[38] In a similar analysis of the evidence in favour of routine mammography for women aged forty to forty-nine, Jane Wells concludes that in 1997 the American National Cancer Institute modified its interpretation of RCT data, as a result of public and political pressure, in order to support such screening.[39] Marcia Meldrum has examined the interpretation of a number of RCTs between 1946 and 1970 and claims that RCT methodology and interpretation is socially constructed and socially determined, and regards the RCT as a device employed by particular workers to construct a claim of scientific objectivity for their activity.[40]

RCT methodology, then, has continued to undergo modifications since 1948. The conduct of an RCT and the interpretation of its results are socially and politically constructed, and critics continue to attack the scope and function of RCTs. This is all rather reminiscent of the state of play prior to 1948, when the MRC was exploiting the rhetoric of the 'controlled trial' to promote its own work in the face of criticism and opposition. The rhetorical associations did not end in 1948, however, and are powerful and relevant today. Prior to the MRC's publication of its streptomycin trial in 1948, it lumped its various trial methodologies under the label 'controlled'. Such a 'controlled trial' did not designate a single methodology, but signified approval for a trial conducted under the proper supervision and regulation of the MRC and which should therefore, by implication, be regarded as trustworthy and reliable. The MRC nevertheless referred to its 'controlled trials' as if the term *did* refer to a distinct entity. In this sense, the 'controlled trial' was a construct prior to its methodology being codified in 1948. Crucially, however, the rhetorical power and effect of the term 'controlled trial' changed little after 1948. The streptomycin trial codified RCT methodology, and embedded – and in some respects, enhanced – the principal rhetorical associations of the term 'controlled'.

The current rhetoric of control

An analysis of the rhetorical function of the term 'controlled trial' in current discourse is outside the scope of this work, but a few examples might serve to illustrate the fact that the term is ubiquitous in lay use, besides medical and scientific writing. Strictly speaking, in twenty-first century parlance, the phrase 'randomised controlled trial' is tautologous. 'Controlled', in its technical meaning, refers to the presence of an untreated, or differently-treated, comparison group. But the presence of such a comparison group is implicit in the description of the trial as 'randomised', since this refers specifically to the random allocation of subjects into different groups in order to receive, or not receive, the therapy under investigation; and nowadays, few trials would contemplate a comparison group without such random allocation. A description of a trial simply as 'randomised' should suffice – indeed, the current issue of the influential *Oxford Textbook of Medicine* employs the term 'randomized trial' in its account of evidence-based medicine.[41]

However 'controlled' will not die and the description of therapeutic trials as 'controlled' remains commonplace. The term is ubiquitous in medical writing, but newspapers, radio and TV also frequently emphasise the 'controlled' nature of evidence favouring, or opposing, a therapy, particularly when controversy surrounds the treatment in question. Assessing the effectiveness of Chinese herbal medicine, the *Daily Mail* advises its readers that there are 'few scientific trials to show that it works. However, a controlled trial carried out at North London's Royal Free Hospital showed that Chinese herbs helped treat 60 per cent of patients suffering from eczema.'[42] The author of this article did not define a 'controlled trial', but to use the term in juxtaposition with the statement that 'there are few scientific trials' implies that the 'controlled' status of this trial carries scientific respectability. The presence or absence of a comparison group is not mentioned. Similarly, in an examination of the evidence supporting a commercially-available allergy test the *Daily Mail* suggests that 'more clinically controlled trials'[43] are required to establish its usefulness. 'Clinically controlled trial' is not defined and is not a phrase which would be familiar to any medical researcher – not a problem, since it appears in an article for the lay reader – but it does beg the question as to what the writer intended to convey. Not, apparently, a trial which necessarily employs a comparison group; rather, perhaps, one possessing a degree of scientific rigour and establishment acceptability.

Phil Barker bemoans in *The Guardian* the paucity of 'rigorously controlled trials of ECT' which, he considers, 'reflects badly on the scientific pretensions of psychiatric medicine.'[44] 'Rigorously controlled' trials are, he implies, a prerequisite before one can aspire to scientific pretensions; again, the meaning of this phrase is not defined, but it seems unlikely that the rigour for which the writer is calling refers solely to the careful allocation of comparison and treatment subjects. Rather, the phrase 'rigorously controlled' offers a rhetorical stamp of scientific respectability. In another *Guardian* article, Jenni Russell awaits 'controlled trials on humans'[45] to establish whether the chemical acrylamide is carcinogenic; Jerome Burne, also writing in *The Guardian*, notes that 'one small *but controlled* trial'[46] has shown that the drug Ampligen appears to be effective in the treatment of chronic fatigue syndrome. The actress Jane Asher makes a plea for animal experiments, arguing that 'carefully controlled, humanely conducted experiments'[47] are unobjectionable; Celia Hall, medical editor of the *Daily Telegraph*, concludes that antenatal screening tests for Down's syndrome do not work in real life 'outside carefully controlled and monitored clinical trials;'[48] another *Daily Telegraph* health correspondent warns that a 'controlled study of 300 people'[49] suggests that indigestion remedies might predispose individuals to food allergies.

In none of these instances do the writers appear to intend 'controlled' to convey the presence of comparison subjects in a trial. Rather, the word appears to serve predominantly to endorse the scientific credentials of a piece of evidence. This impression is reinforced by the frequency with which the word 'controlled' is used with a qualifying adverb, 'carefully controlled', 'rigorously controlled', 'clinically controlled'. Such qualifiers should have little or nothing to add to the technical meaning of 'controlled' as a study possessing a comparison group, but they contribute substantially to the term's rhetorical impact.

Possibly these writers are simply sloppy, or do not know, or care, what is the current technical meaning of a 'controlled' trial. This is, however, an unlikely explanation for the widespread use of the term. Writers with a lay readership can, and do, employ the technical meaning of 'controlled' on occasions when it suits them – for example, Wendy Moore puzzles in *The Observer* why doctors cannot prescribe placebos 'except in carefully controlled trials',[50] and Roger Highfield describes in the *Daily Telegraph* how a doctor investigating brain tissue implants in the treatment of Parkinson's disease 'designed a controlled trial by taking the controversial step of including a placebo group who had "sham surgery", holes drilled into their skulls but no tissue implanted.'[51]

The 'controlled trial' to which these writers refer, represents just as much a rhetorical construct as the MRC's 'controlled trial' prior to 1948 – an idealised, scientifically valid, establishment-approved endeavour. The RCT is, and always has been, one of a number of available methodologies for assessing therapeutic efficacy. It achieved, and maintains, its current hegemonic position partly through the rhetorical power of its 'controlled' status. This argument is by no means intended to deprive the RCT of any authority – given current understanding of the nature of health and disease and of the mechanism of action of treatment modalities, the RCT is by general consensus the most appropriate tool for the large part of therapeutic assessment. But there are other methodologies – observational studies,[52] case reports,[53] 'computrials'[54] – whose advocates feel they have been rather left out in the cold.

Rhetoric in evidence-based medicine

The rhetorical associations of the term 'controlled' remain relevant to the current discourse within EBM, but 'controlled' is one word within a field which appears well stocked with potentially powerful rhetorical terms. Indeed, some commentators prefer to view the entire EBM enterprise as fundamentally a rhetorical endeavour. George Weisz suggests that EBM is likely increasingly to be employed as a rhetorical device to enhance medical authority,[55] in an argument reminiscent of commentators such as Toth, Cox, and Meldrum (see Chapter 1) who make similar claims for the RCT. Andrew Van de Ven and Margaret Schomaker[56] examine EBM against the background of Aristotle's system of rhetoric, whereby an argument consists of three parts – *logos*, the logic of the message; *pathos*, the argument's emotional appeal to the audience; and *ethos*, the authority and credibility of the speaker. An argument necessarily consists of all three components, a notion sometimes lost upon proponents of EBM who too easily assume that their logos alone will win the day. Clinicians' use of EBM in practice is also substantially rhetorical; although the British doctors in Louise Fitzgerald and Sue Dopson's analyses claimed to be influenced primarily by evidence from RCTs in making therapeutic decisions, in actual fact they adopted various alternative notions of 'evidence', particularly the tacit knowledge and experience of senior colleagues.[57] Studies by clinicians and medical sociologists have demonstrated that practitioners – even those with an avowed commitment to evidence-based practice – are influenced by factors such as experience, anecdote, rationale, and even intuition, besides published RCT data, when they make real treatment decisions in practice.[58] Doctors are less likely to prescribe warfarin, a drug to inhibit blood clotting, if they have encountered a patient who had suffered the side-effect of a serious bleed;[59] early memories from hospital training influence GPs practice years later;[60] and doctors who are aware of the RCT evidence regarding the choice of antidepressant medication nevertheless make treatment decisions according to their perception of the particular needs of the patient before them.[61] Stefan Timmermans and Marc Berg examined EBM in practice amongst one group of junior hospital residents in a United States hospital with a declared commitment to EBM. Despite the rhetoric of EBM, 'evidence' in practice frequently comprised the opinions of senior clinicians in the hospital hierarchy. Some junior doctors – tagged 'librarians' in Timmermans and Berg's analysis – regarded almost any written source as authoritative evidence, in contrast to 'researcher' doctors who were more able to approach RCTs critically.[62]

'Evidence', then, appears to be a hazier concept than some proponents of EBM would suggest. In practice, the notion includes experience, the opinions of colleagues and superiors, personal beliefs, and the perceived needs of individual patients besides published data from trials, systematic reviews, and meta-analyses. Even such published data – the 'hardest' evidence which occupies the top of the EBM hierarchy – is subject to interpretation and social negotiation. The potential for differing interpretations of RCTs is discussed above; the same process attaches to meta-analysis and systematic review. Meta-analysis takes a leap of faith by assuming that results from several different studies can be combined and analysed as if they were one large study; the statistical trickery required to achieve this has led to the technique being described as 'statistical alchemy' by the influential EBM commentator Alvan Feinstein.[63] 'The evidence' from RCTs does not simply speak for itself, even when it is being aggregated or assessed for meta-analysis or systematic review – otherwise why would different meta-analyses and systematic reviews relating to the same subject, reach such different conclusions?[64]

Evidence means different things to different practitioners; it can mean different things to the same practitioner, even at the same time; it involves negotiation, interpretation, and social networks.[65] Evidence becomes a construct. Sue Dopson and Louise Fitzgerald are investigators of organisational systems; in their analysis of a number of studies into the incorporation of EBM into practice they conclude: 'There is no such thing as 'the evidence', there are simply bodies of evidence.... The available bodies of evidence are socially and historically constructed.'[66] Like the controlled trial in the early-twentieth century, evidence is a construct, and like the controlled trial, the term 'evidence' enjoys considerable rhetorical power. Evidence can sway the decision of a court of law, can send a miscreant to jail, or set the innocent free. Who can argue with evidence? How potent is the orator who claims evidence on his side!

Jeanne Daly argues that adherents of EBM have colonised the very meaning of the term 'evidence' to include only the upper reaches of their own hierarchy of evidence, primarily RCTs.[67] This is a process apparently similar to the colonisation of the term 'controlled' by the MRC during the early-twentieth century, for which I have argued in this work. Just as a therapeutic trial becomes unthinkable if it is not 'controlled' – whatever that means – therapeutic decisions become unreliable unless they are based upon 'evidence', implying specifically one narrowly-defined notion of evidence. One group of commentators has even denounced the EBM movement as 'fascist' for its exclusion of other forms of knowledge-making and evidence.[68]

My intention is not to weigh in against EBM as the most pragmatic philosophy to enable therapeutic practice which is most likely to achieve positive results, nor is it to attempt to knock the RCT off its perch as currently the most effective means to evaluate a therapy. But just as the rhetorical exploitation of the term 'controlled' helped the RCT achieve, and still helps it to maintain, its position at the top of the hierarchy of evidence, similar forces appear to be at work in persuading us of the unassailable sanctity of 'evidence.'

Notes

1. Fragile varicose veins inside the oesophagus (gullet) which can be prone to profuse, and frequently fatal, bleeding
2. I.M. Macintyre, 'Tribulations for Clinical Trials', *British Medical Journal,* 302 (1991), 1099–100.
3. B. Haynes, 'Can it Work? Does it Work? Is it Worth it?', *British Medical Journal,* 319 (1999), 652–3.
4. *Ibid.*
5. Council for International Organizations of Medical Sciences, *Controlled Clinical Trials: Papers Delivered at the Conference Convened by the Council for International Organizations of Medical Sciences* (Oxford: Blackwell, 1960).
6. H. Atkins, 'Conduct of a Controlled Clinical Trial', *British Medical Journal* 2 (1966), 377–9.
7. *Ibid.,* 377.
8. I. Chalmers, C. Rounding and K. Lock, 'Descriptive Survey of Non-Commercial Randomised Controlled Trials in the United Kingdom, 1980–2002', *British Medical Journal* 327 (2003), 1017–20; T. Fahey *et al.,* 'The Type and Quality of Randomized Controlled Trials (RCTs) Published in UK Public Health Journals', *Journal of Public Health Medicine,* 17, 4 (1995), 469–74; R.H. Fletcher and S.W. Fletcher, 'Clinical Research in General Medical Journals: A 30-Year Perspective', *New England Journal of Medicine* 301, 4 (1979), 180–3; M.M. McDermott *et al.,* 'Changes in Study Design, Gender Issues, and other Characteristics of Clinical Research Published in Three Major Medical Journals from 1971 to 1991', *Journal of General Internal Medicine* 10, 1 (1995), 13–18; S. McDonald *et al.* and the Cochrane Centres' Working Group on 50 years of Randomized Trials. 'Number and Size of Randomized Trials Reported in General Health Care Journals from 1948 to 1997', *International Journal of Epidemiology* 31 (2002), 125–7; C.A. Silagy and D. Jewell, 'Review of 39 Years of Randomized Controlled Trials in the British Journal of General Practice', *British Journal of General Practice,* 44 (1994), 359–63.
9. McDonald *et al., ibid.*
10. *Ibid.*
11. C. Ceballos et al., 'Why Evidence-Based Medicine? 20 Years of Meta-Analysis', *Anales de Medicina Interna,* 17, 10 (2000), 521–6. (Spanish article, English abstract).
12. G.J. Kutcher, *Clinical Ethics and Research Imperatives in Human Experiments: A Case of Contested Knowledge* (PhD thesis: Cambridge University, 2001); J.R. Matthews, *Quantification and the Quest for Medical Certainty* (Princeton: Princeton University Press, 1995); S. Timmermans and M. Berg, 'Standardizing Risk' in S. Timmermans and M. Berg, *The Gold Standard:*

The Challenge of Evidence-Based Medicine and Standardization in Health Care
(Philadelphia: Temple University Press, 2003), 166–94.

13. T.M. Porter, *Trust in Numbers: Objectivity in Science and Public Life*
(Princeton: Princeton University Press, 1995); a number of commentators
accept Porter's reasoning, see for example, Ilana Löwy, *Between Bench and
Bedside: Science, Healing and Interleukin-2 in a Cancer Ward* (Cambridge:
Harvard University Press, 1996), see 48–54; also Timmermans and Berg,
ibid., 138–9.

14. H.M. Marks, *The Progress of Experiment: Science and Therapeutic Reform in
the United States, 1900–1990* (Cambridge: Cambridge University Press,
1997).

15. J. Daly, *Evidence-Based Medicine and the Search for a Science of Clinical Care*
(Berkeley: University of California Press, 2005), 15–16.

16. I. Chalmers, 'Unbiased, Relevant, and Reliable Assessments in Health Care',
British Medical Journal, 317 (1998), 1167–8.

17. I. Russell, 'Evaluating New Surgical Procedures', *British Medical Journal,* 311
(1995), 1243–4; P.F. Ridgway and A.W. Darzi, 'Placebos and Standardising
New Surgical Techniques', *British Medical Journal,* 325 (2002), 560.

18. J. Clark, 'Preventive Home Visits to Elderly People', *British Medical Journal,*
323 (2001), 708.

19. A.G. Sutcliffe, 'Prescribing Medicines for Children', *British Medical Journal,*
319 (1999), 70–1; R. Smith, 'Babies and Consent: Yet Another NHS
Scandal', *British Medical Journal,* 320 (2000), 1285–6.

20. S.J.L. Edwards, R.J. Lilford and J. Hewison, 'The Ethics of Randomised
Controlled Trials from the Perspectives of Patients, the Public and Healthcare
Professionals', *British Medical Journal,* 317 (1998), 1209–12.

21. K. Featherstone and J. Donovan, 'Random Allocation or Allocation at
Random? Patients' Perspectives of Participation in a Randomised Controlled
Trial', *British Medical Journal,* 317 (1998), 1177–80.

22. A.J. Welton *et al.*, 'Is Recruitment More Difficult with a Placebo Arm in
Randomised Controlled Trials? A Quasirandomised, Interview Based Study',
British Medical Journal, 318 (1999), 1114–17.

23. E. Richards, *Vitamin C and Cancer: Medicine or Politics?* (Basingstoke:
Macmillan, 1991).

24. S. Epstein, *Impure Science: AIDS, Activism, and the Politics of Knowledge*
(Berkeley: University of California Press, 1996).

25. M.D. Sullivan, 'Placebo Controls and Epistemic Control in Orthodox
Medicine', *Journal of Medical Philosophy,* 18, 2 (1993), 213–31.

26. K. Fairhurst and C. Dowrick, 'Problems with Recruitment in a Randomized
Controlled Trial of Counselling in General Practice: Causes and
Implications', *Journal of Health Service Research* 1, 2 (1996), 77–80; D. Van
der Windt *et al.*, 'Practical Aspects of Conducting a Pragmatic Randomised

182

Trial in Primary Care: Patient Recruitment and Outcome Assessment',
British Journal of General Practice, 50 (2000), 371–4.

27. A.C. Freeman and K. Sweeney, 'Why General Practitioners do not
Implement Evidence: Qualitative Study', *British Medical Journal,* 323
(2001), 1100–2.

28. D. Torgerson and B. Sibbald, 'Understanding Controlled Trials: What is a
Patient Preference Trial?', *British Medical Journal,* 316 (1998), 360.

29. A. Sheikh, L. Smeeth and R. Ashcroft, 'Randomised Controlled Trials in
Primary Care: Scope and Application', *British Journal of General Practice* 52
(2002), 746–51.

30. *Ibid.*

31. P. Hawe, A. Shiell and T. Riley, 'Complex Interventions: How "Out of
Control" can a Randomised Controlled Trial be?', *British Medical Journal,*
328 (2004), 1561–3.

32. L. Cranberg, 'Evaluating New Treatments', *British Medical Journal,* 317
(1998), 1260.

33. J. Concato, N. Shah and R. Horwitz, 'Randomized, Controlled Trials,
Observational Studies, and the Hierarchy of Research Designs', *New England
Journal of Medicine,* 342 (2000), 1887–92.

34. This is a widely discussed argument; see for example, K. Sweeney, 'Personal
Knowledge', *British Medical Journal* ,332 (2006), 129–30; Daly, *op. cit.* (note
15), particularly chapter 9; G. Weisz, 'From Clinical Counting to Evidence-
Based Medicine', in G. Jorland, A. Opinel and G. Weisz (eds.), *Body Counts:
Medical Quantification in Historical and Sociological Perspective* (Montreal:
McGill-Queen's University Press, 2005), 377–93.

35. R. Peto and C. Baigent, 'Trials: The Next Fifty Years', *British Medical
Journal,* 317 (1998), 1170–1.

36. Richards, *op. cit.* (note 23), 6.

37. *Ibid.,* 233.

38. J. McCormack and T. Greenhalgh, 'Seeing What You Want to See in
Randomised Controlled Trials: Versions and Perversions of UKPDS Data',
British Medical Journal, 320 (2000), 1720–3.

39. J. Wells, 'Mammography and the Politics of Randomised Controlled Trials',
British Medical Journal, 317 (1998), 1224–30.

40. M. Meldrum, *"Departures from Design": The Randomized Clinical Trial in
Historical Context, 1946–1970* (PhD thesis: State University of New York at
Stony Brook, 1994), 373.

41. R. Collins *et al.,* 'Large-Scale Randomized Evidence: Trials and Overviews',
in D. Warrell *et al.,* (eds), *Oxford Textbook of Medicine, Volume 1,* 4th edn
(Oxford, Oxford University Press, 2003), 24–36.

42. N. Coleman, 'How Acupuncture and Herbal Medicine can Heal your Body',
Daily Mail (Health section), 31 January 2003.

43. N. Coleman, 'More Allergy Tests under the Microscope', *Daily Mail* (Women & Family Section), 30 May 2002.

44. P. Barker, 'Shock Tactics', *The Guardian,* 9 May 2003.

45. J. Russell, 'Could These Foods be Giving Us Cancer?' *The Guardian,* 15 August 2002.

46. J. Burne, 'Battle Fatigue', *The Guardian,* 30 March 2002, (my italics).

47. D. Derbyshire, 'Asher Makes the Case for Animal Experiments', *Daily Telegraph,* 9 October 2003.

48. C. Hall, 'New Down's Tests are Disappointing', *Daily Telegraph,* 5 July 2002.

49. M. Day, 'Anti-Indigestion Pills Blamed for Food Allergy Cases', *Daily Telegraph,* 28 September 2003.

50. W. Moore, 'Faith Healing', *The Observer,* 15 December 2002.

51. R. Highfield, 'Parkinson's Sufferers "Worse" after Transplants', *Daily Telegraph,* 14 March 2001.

52. Concato, Shah and Horwitz, *op. cit.* (note 33).

53. T. Greenhalgh and B. Hurwitz, 'Narrative Based Medicine: Why Study Narrative?' *British Medical Journal,* 318 (1999), 48–50; I.R. McEwen, 'Case Reports: Slices of Real Life to Complement Evidence', *Physical Therapy,* 84 (2004), 126–7.

54. Cranberg, *op. cit.* (note 32).

55. Weisz, *op. cit.* (note 34).

56. A. Van de Ven and M. Schomaker, 'The Rhetoric of Evidence-Based Medicine', *Health Care Management Review* 27, 3 (2002), 89–91.

57. L. Fitzgerald and S. Dopson, 'Knowledge, Credible Evidence, and Utilization', in S. Dopson and L. Fitzgerald (eds), *Knowledge to Action? Evidence-Based Health Care in Context* (Oxford: Oxford University Press, 2005), 132–54.

58. Sweeney, *op. cit.* (note 34); T. Greenhalgh, 'Intuition and Evidence: Uneasy Bedfellows?', *British Journal of General Practice* 52 (2002), 395–400.

59. N.K. Choudhry *et al.,* 'Impact of Adverse Events on Prescribing Warfarin in Patients with Atrial Fibrillation: Matched Pair Analysis', *British Medical Journal,* 332 (2006), 141–3.

60. Freeman and Sweeney, *op. cit.* (note 27).

61. D. Armstrong, 'Clinical Autonomy, Individual and Collective: The Problem of Changing Doctors' Behaviour', *Social Science and Medicine,* 55 (2002), 1771–7.

62. Timmermans and Berg, 'Evidence-Based Medicine and Learning to Doctor' in *op. cit.* (note 12), 142–65.

63. A. Feinstein, 'Meta-Analysis: Statistical Alchemy for the 21st Century', *Journal of Clinical Epidemiology,* 48, 1 (1995), 71–9.

64. G.G.L. Biondi-Zoccai et al., 'Compliance with QUOROM and Quality of Reporting of Overlapping Meta-Analyses on the Role of Acetylcysteine in

the Prevention of Contrast Associated Nephropathy: Case Study', *British Medical Journal*, 332 (2006), 202–6; T.C. Chalmers *et al.*, 'Meta-Analysis of Clinical Trials as a Scientific Discipline. 11: Replicate Variability and Comparison of Studies that Agree and Disagree', *Statistics in Medicine* 6, 7 (1987), 733–44; A.R. Jadad *et al.*, 'Systematic Reviews and Meta-Analyses on Treatment of Asthma: Critical Evaluation', *British Medical Journal*, 320 (2000), 537–40.

65. For a further development of this theme see S. Dopson and L. Fitzgerald (eds), *Knowledge to Action? Evidence-Based Health Care in Context* (Oxford: Oxford University Press, 2005).

66. Fitzgerald and Dopson, *op. cit.* (note 57), 139.

67. Daly, *op. cit.* (note 15), 231.

68. D. Holmes *et al.*, 'Deconstructing the Evidence-Based Discourse in Health Sciences: Truth, Power and Fascism', *International Journal of Evidence-Based Healthcare* 4, 3 (2006), 180–6.

Bibliography

Primary sources

Editorials [Journal/Date]

Editorial, 'Sherwood Colliery U-V-R', *British Journal of Actinotherapy*, 3 (1928), 42–3.

Editorial, 'The Colebrook Report', *British Journal of Actinotherapy and Physiotherapy*, 4 (1929), 134.

Editorial, 'The M.R.C. Report, 1928–29', *British Journal of Actinotherapy and Physiotherapy*, 5 (1930), 1–2.

Editorial, 'Insulin and Diabetes', *British Medical Journal*, ii (1922), 882.

Editorial, 'The Treatment of Diabetes by Insulin', *British Medical Journal*, ii (1922), 991–2.

Editorial, 'The Price of Insulin', *British Medical Journal*, i (1924), 339.

Editorial, 'The Medical Research Council', *British Medical Journal*, i (1925), 225–6.

Editorial, 'Dangers of Ultra-Violet Light Baths', *British Medical Journal*, i (1925), 708.

Editorial, 'Glandular Therapy', *British Medical Journal*, i (1925), 1137.

Editorial, 'Light and Health', *British Medical Journal*, ii (1925), 525–6.

Editorial, 'Photosynthesis and the Origin of Vitamins', *British Medical Journal*, ii (1925), 961.

Editorial, 'Artificial Light Clinics in Glasgow', *British Medical Journal*, i (1926), 494–5.

Editorial, 'Auto-Experimenters', *British Medical Journal*, i (1926), 914.

Editorial, 'The Popular Lecture', *British Medical Journal*, ii (1926), 211.

Editorial, 'Light Therapy and Immunity', *British Medical Journal*, i (1928), 362–3.

Bibliography

Editorial, 'Actinotherapy: The Need for Control', *British Medical Journal,* ii (1928), 661–2.

Editorial, 'Electrocution from Ultra-Violet Ray Lamp', *British Medical Journal,* i (1929), 163.

Editorial, 'Actinotherapy', *British Medical Journal,* i (1929), 562–3.

Editorial, 'Therapeutic Effects of Ultra-Violet Irradiation', *British Medical Journal,* ii (1929), 585–6.

Editorial, 'Sulphanilamide in Urinary Infections', *British Medical Journal,* ii (1937), 589–90.

Editorial, 'Sir Almroth Wright', *British Medical Journal,* i (1947), 646–7.

Editorial, 'Streptomycin in Pulmonary Tuberculosis', *British Medical Journal,* ii (1948), 791–2.

Editorial, 'The Controlled Therapeutic Trial', *British Medical Journal,* ii (1948), 791–2.

Editorial, 'The Prevention of Influenza', *British Medical Journal,* ii (1953), 1206–7.

Editorial, 'Out, Damned Spot', *British Medical Journal,* ii (1951), 1074–5.

Editorial, 'The Administration of Insulin', *Journal of the American Medical Association,* 81 (1923), 753.

Editorial, 'Can Insulin Replace the Pancreas?' *Journal of the American Medical Association,* 84 (1925), 1122.

Editorial, 'Sun-Worship', *Lancet,* i (1929), 615–6.

Editorial, 'The Treatment of Diabetes by Insulin', *Lancet,* i (1923), 391–2.

Editorial Annotation, 'Serum Treatment of Pneumonia', *Lancet,* i (1930), 30–1.

Editorial, 'Oral Anti-Diabetic Remedies', *Lancet,* i (1931), 31–2.

Editorial Annotations, 'Clinical Trials of New Remedies', *Lancet,* ii (1931), 304.

Editorial, 'Influenza B', *Lancet,* ii (1946), 644.

Obituaries [subject]

Obituary, 'Sir Christopher Andrewes', *British Medical Journal,* 298 (1989), 180.

Obituary, 'Richard Armstrong', *British Medical Journal,* 2 (1975), 44.

Obituary, 'Dora C. Colebrook', *British Medical Journal,* 1 (1966), 174–5.

Bibliography

Obituary, 'Sir Walter Fletcher', *British Medical Journal*, i (1933), 1085.

Obituary, 'Sir Francis Fraser', *British Medical Journal*, ii (1964), 950–1.

Obituary, 'George Graham', *British Medical Journal*, 4 (1971), 563.

Obituary, 'Sir Austin Bradford Hill', *British Medical Journal*, 302 (1991), 1017.

Obituary, 'Sir Patrick Laidlaw', *British Medical Journal*, i (1940), 551–2.

Obituary, 'Robert Lawrence', *British Medical Journal*, 3 (1968), 621–2.

Obituary, 'R.L. Mackenzie Wallis', *British Medical Journal*, i (1929), 710–11.

Obituary, 'D. Murray Lyon', *British Medical Journal*, ii (1956), 1309–10.

Obituary, 'E. Sharpey-Schafer', *The Fight Against Disease* XXIII, 2 (1935), 22–5.

Obituary, 'Wilson Smith', *British Medical Journal*, ii (1965), 240.

Obituary, 'Charles Stuart-Harris', *British Medical Journal*, 314 (1997), 906–7.

Obituary, 'Sir Harold Whittingham', *British Medical Journal*, 287 (1983), 369.

Obituary, 'Almroth Edward Wright', *Lancet*, i (1947), 654–6.

Obituary, 'Sir Almroth Wright', *British Medical Journal*, i (1947), 657–8.

Authored Articles and Books [Author/Title]

C.R. Affleck, 'Raw Pancreas by the Mouth in the Treatment of Diabetes', *British Medical Journal*, i (1926), 727.

G.A. Allan, 'Diabetes Mellitus and its Treatment by Insulin', *British Medical Journal*, i (1924), 50–3.

J.M. Alston and J.G. McCrie, 'Concentrated Antipneumococcal Serum in the Treatment of Lobar Pneumonia', *British Medical Journal*, i (1931), 817–8.

American Medical Association, *Glandular Therapy* (Chicago: American Medical Association, 1925).

T. Anderson, 'Sulphanilamide in the Treatment of Measles', *British Medical Journal*, i (1937), 716–18.

J.C. Appleby, F. Himmelweit and C.H. Stuart-Harris, 'Immunisation with Influenza Virus A Vaccines: Comparison of Intradermal and Subcutaneous Routes', *Lancet*, 1 (1951), 1384–7.

R.R. Armstrong and R.S. Johnson, 'Concentrated Antipneumococcal Serum in the Treatment of Lobar Pneumonia', *British Medical Journal*, i (1931), 701–2.

Bibliography

R.R. Armstrong, and R.S. Johnson, 'Homologous Antipneumocooccal Serums in the Treatment of Lobar Pneumonia', *British Medical Journal*, i (1931), 931–6.

R.R. Armstrong, 'Immediate Pneumococcal Typing', *British Medical Journal*, i (1932), 187–8.

R.R. Armstrong, 'Immediate Pneumococcal Typing', *British Medical Journal*, i (1932), 260.

R.R. Armstrong, 'A Swift and Simple Method for Deciding Pneumococcal "Type"', *British Medical Journal*, i (1931), 241–5.

J.N. Badham, 'More Blasts on the Trumpet', *British Medical Journal*, ii (1951), 1218.

H.S. Banks, 'Chemotherapy of Meningococcal Meningitis', *Lancet*, ii (1939), 921–6.

H.S. Banks, 'Therapeutic Value of Ultra-Violet Light', *British Medical Journal*, i (1929), 662.

A.S. Barr, 'More Blasts on the Trumpet', *British Medical Journal*, ii (1951), 1218–9.

R.H. Beckett, *Modern Actinotherapy* (London: William Heinemann Medical, 1955), 1–6.

J. Bernstein, 'Raw Pancreas by Mouth Compared with Insulin', *British Medical Journal*, ii (1925), 844.

J. Bernstein, 'Raw Pancreas by Mouth Compared with Insulin', *British Medical Journal*, ii (1925), 979.

W. Broadbent, 'Reports of Societies: The Treatment of Pneumonia', *British Medical Journal*, i (1931), 446–8.

J. Brown, 'Influence of Sunlight and Artificial Light on Health', *British Medical Journal*, ii (1925), 477.

J. Burne, 'Battle Fatigue', *The Guardian*, 30 March 2002.

P.J. Cammidge, 'The Effects of Pancreas Preparations by the Mouth upon Carbohydrate Metabolism', *British Medical Journal*, ii (1925), 1216–8.

P.J. Cammidge, 'Treatment of Diabetes by Raw Fresh Gland (Pancreas)', *British Medical Journal*, i (1925), 805.

D.W. Carmalt-Jones, 'Sir Almroth Wright', *Lancet*, i (1947), 930.

R. Carrasco-Formiguera, 'Treatment of Diabetes by Raw Fresh Gland (Pancreas)', *British Medical Journal*, ii (1925), 552–3.

Bibliography

R. Cecil, 'Serum Treatment of Pneumonia', *British Medical Journal*, ii (1932), 263.

N.K. Choudhry, G.M. Anderson, A. Laupacis, D. Ross-Degnan, S.-L.T. Normand, and S.B. Soumerai, 'Impact of Adverse Events on Prescribing Warfarin in Patients with Atrial Fibrillation: Matched Pair Analysis', *British Medical Journal*, 332 (2006), 141–3.

J.B. Christopherson and M. Broadbent, 'Ephedrine and Pseudo-Ephedrine in Asthma, Bronchial Asthma, and Enuresis', *British Medical Journal*, i (1934), 978–9.

S. Churchill, 'Treatment by Light', *The Guardian,* 30 September 1929.

A.J. Clark, 'The Experimental Basis of Endocrine Therapy', *British Medical Journal*, ii (1923), 51–3.

J. Clark, 'Preventive Home Visits to Elderly People', *British Medical Journal*, 323 (2001), 708.

D. Colebrook, *Artificial Sunlight in Industry* (London: HMSO, 1946).

D. Colebrook, 'Debate on Actinotherapy', *British Medical Journal*, i (1930), 150.

D. Colebrook, *Irradiation and Health* (London: HMSO, 1929).

D. Colebrook, 'Varicose Ulcers: A Comparison of Treatment by Ultra-Violet Light and Unna's Paste Dressings', *Lancet*, i (1928), 904–7.

L. Colebrook and A.W. Purdie, 'Treatment of 106 Cases of Puerperal Fever by Sulphanilamide', *Lancet*, ii (1937), 1237–42 and 1291–3.

L. Colebrook, 'Dora Challis Colebrook', *Lancet,* 2 (1965), 1248.

N. Coleman, 'How Acupuncture and Herbal Medicine can Heal your Body', *Daily Mail* (Health section), 31 January 2003.

N. Coleman, 'More Allergy Tests under the Microscope', *Daily Mail* (Women & Family Section), 30 May 2002.

E.L. Collis and M. Greenwood, *The Health of the Industrial Worker* (London: J. and A. Churchill, 1921).

J. Concato, N. Shah and R. Horwitz, 'Randomized, Controlled Trials, Observational Studies, and the Hierarchy of Research Designs', *New England Journal of Medicine*, 342 (2000), 1887–92.

J. Cowan, *et al.*, 'Treatment of Lobar Pneumonia by Felton's Serum', *Lancet,* ii (1930), 1387–90.

W.N. Cowles, 'A Case of Diabetes Treated by Feeding of Calves' Pancreas', *Boston Medical and Surgical Journal*, 74 (1911), 921–2.

Bibliography

L. Cranberg, 'Evaluating New Treatments', *British Medical Journal,* 317 (1998), 1260.

S.L. Cummins, 'Merthiolate in the Treatment of Tuberculosis', *Lancet,* ii (1937), 962–3.

H.H. Dale, 'Almroth Edward Wright', *British Medical Journal,* i (1947), 659.

H.H. Dale, 'A Lecture on the Physiology of Insulin', *Lancet,* i (1923), 989–93.

H.H. Dale, 'Sir Walter Fletcher', *British Medical Journal,* i (1933), 1085–6.

C. Dalton, 'Ultra-Violet Ray Therapy', *British Medical Journal,* ii (1928), 821.

Lord Dawson of Penn, 'The Treatment of Lobar Pneumonia', *Lancet,* i (1931), 625–7.

Lord Dawson of Penn, 'The Treatment of Pneumonia', *British Medical Journal,* i (1931), 446–8.

M. Day, 'Anti-Indigestion Pills Blamed for Food Allergy Cases', *Daily Telegraph,* 28 September 2003.

D. Derbyshire, 'Asher Makes the Case for Animal Experiments', *Daily Telegraph,* 9 October 2003.

W.E. Dixon, 'The Therapeutic Value of Light', *British Medical Journal,* ii (1925), 499–500.

R. Doll and A.B. Hill, 'The Mortality of Doctors in Relation to their Smoking Habits', *British Medical Journal,* i (1954), 1451–5

R. Doll, 'Austin Bradford Hill', *Lancet,* 337 (1991), 1154.

R. Doll, 'Austin Bradford Hill', *Biographical Memoirs of Fellows of the Royal Society,* 40 (1994), 129–40.

R. Doll, 'Sir Austin Bradford Hill and the Progress of Medical Science', *British Medical Journal,* 305 (1992), 1521–6.

S.E. Dore, 'The Uses and Limitations of Ultra-Violet Radiation in Dermatology', *British Medical Journal,* ii (1927), 255–7.

S.E. Dore, 'Uses and Limitations of Ultra-Violet Radiation Therapy', *British Medical Journal,* i (1927), 565.

J.A. Dudgeon, *et al.,* 'Influenza B in 1945-46', *Lancet,* 2 (1946), 627–31.

W. Dunn, 'Treatment of Diabetes by Raw Fresh Gland (Pancreas)', *British Medical Journal,* i (1925), 680.

Edinburgh Royal Infirmary [Physicians to the], 'A Report on Lobar Pneumonia Treated by Concentrated Antiserum', *Lancet,* ii (1930), 1390–94.

Editors of the British Medical Journal, *The Endocrines in Theory and Practice: Articles Republished from the British Medical Journal.* (London : H.K. Lewis, 1937).

A. Eidinow, 'Actinotherapy', *British Medical Journal,* ii (1925), 71.

W.D. Emery, 'Vaccine Therapy', in A.E. Wright (ed.), *Vaccine Therapy, its Administration, Value and Limitations: A Discussion Opened by Sir Almroth E. Wright* (London: Longmans, Green & Co., 1910), 187–97.

J.W. Eyre, 'Vaccine Therapy', in A.E. Wright, *Vaccine Therapy, its Administration, Value and Limitations* (London: Longmans, Green & Co., 1910), 60–4.

K. Fairhurst and C. Dowrick, 'Problems with Recruitment in a Randomized Controlled Trial of Counselling in General Practice: Causes and Implications', *Journal of Health Service Research* 1, 2 (1996), 77–80.

K. Featherstone and J. Donovan, 'Random Allocation or Allocation at Random? Patients' Perspectives of Participation in a Randomised Controlled Trial', *British Medical Journal,* 317 (1998), 1177–80.

A. Fleming and G.F. Petrie, *Recent Advances in Vaccine and Serum Therapy* (Philadelphia: P. Blakiston's Son & Co. Inc., 1934), 125.

W. Fletcher, 'An Address on the Scope and Needs of Medical Research', *British Medical Journal,* ii (1932), 43–7.

W. Fletcher, 'Royal Dental Hospital: Address', *British Medical Journal,* ii (1927), 655–6.

R. Fisher, *The Design of Experiments* (Edinburgh: Oliver and Boyd, 1935).

F.T. Ford, E.S. Robinson and R. Heffro, *Chemotherapy and Serum Therapy of Pneumonia* (London: Humphrey Milford, Oxford University Press, 1940).

T. Fox, 'Foreword', in A.B. Hill, *Principles of Medical Statistics,* 1st edn (London: The Lancet, 1937).

J. Freeman, 'Sir Almroth Wright', *British Medical Journal,* i (1947), 659–60.

C.B.S Fuller, 'Oral administration of Pancreatic and Other Preparations in Diabetes', *British Medical Journal,* i (1928), 798–800.

A. Furniss, *Ultra-Violet Therapy: A Compilation of Papers forming a Review of the Subject* (London: William Heinemann, 1931), 1–4.

Bibliography

E. Gehan and N.A. Lemak, *Statistics in Medical Research: Developments in Clinical Trials* (New York: Plenum Medical Book Co., 1994)

E. Glynn and L. Digby, *Bacteriological and Clinical Observations on Pneumonia and Empyemata, with Special Reference to the Pneumococcus and to Serum Treatment*. (London: HMSO, 1923).

G. Graham and C.F. Harris, 'The Treatment of Diabetes Mellitus with Insulin and Carbohydrate Restriction', *Lancet*, i (1923), 1150–3.

G. Graham, 'Treatment of Diabetes by Raw Fresh Gland (Pancreas)', *British Medical Journal*, i (1925), 859–60.

N. Gray Hill, 'The Therapeutic Value of Ultra-Violet Light', *British Medical Journal*, i (1929), 620.

F.H.K. Green, 'The Clinical Evaluation of Remedies', *Lancet*, ii (1954), 1085–90.

M. Greenwood, 'The Statistician and Medical Research', *British Medical Journal*, ii (1948), 467–8.

M. Greenwood, *Experimental Epidemiology* (London: HMSO, 1936).

C. Griffiths, 'Treatment of Diabetes by Raw Fresh Gland (Pancreas)', *British Medical Journal*, i (1925), 921.

J.A. Gunn, 'Remarks on the Outlook of Research on Therapeutics', *British Medical Journal*, ii (1932), 389–92.

C. Hall, 'New Down's Tests are Disappointing', *Daily Telegraph*, 5 July 2002.

P. Hall, 'Debate on Actinotherapy', *British Medical Journal*, i (1930), 149–50.

P. Hall, 'Individual Overdosage of Ultra-Violet Rays', *British Medical Journal*, i (1926), 349.

P. Hall, 'Ultra-Violet Light', *British Medical Journal*, i (1925), 1061.

G.A. Harrison, 'Can Insulin Produce even a Partial Cure in Human Diabetes Mellitus?', *Quarterly Journal of Medicine*, 19, (1925), 223–34.

G.A. Harrison, 'Treatment of Diabetes by Raw Fresh Gland (Pancreas)', *British Medical Journal*, i (1925), 760–1.

P. Hawe, A. Shiell, and T. Riley, 'Complex Interventions: How "Out of Control" can a Randomised Controlled Trial be?', *British Medical Journal*, 328 (2004), 1561–3.

B. Haynes, 'Can it Work? Does it Work? Is it Worth it?', *British Medical Journal*, 319 (1999), 652–3.

C.B. Heald, 'Abuses of Light Therapy', *Lancet*, i (1928), 392–3.

C.B. Heald, 'Therapeutic Value of Ultra-Violet Light', *British Medical Journal*, i (1929), 744.

R. Highfield, 'Parkinson's Sufferers 'Worse' after Transplants', *Daily Telegraph*, 14 March 2001.

A.B. Hill, 'Aims and Ethics', in Council for International Organizations of Medical Sciences, *Controlled Clinical Trials: Papers Delivered at the Conference Convened by the Council for International Organizations of Medical Sciences* (Oxford: Blackwell, 1960), 3–7.

A.B. Hill, 'The Clinical Trial', *New England Journal of Medicine*, 247, 4 (1952), 113–19.

A.B. Hill, 'Conclusion: The Statistician', in Council for International Organizations of Medical Sciences, *Controlled Clinical Trials: Papers Delivered at the Conference Convened by the Council for International Organizations of Medical Sciences* (Oxford: Blackwell, 1960), 168–71.

A.B. Hill, 'Introduction', in M. Greenwood, *The Medical Dictator and other Biographical Studies* (London: Keynes Press, 1986), xi.

A.B. Hill, 'Medical Ethics and Controlled Trials', *British Medical Journal*, i (1963), 1043–9, 1045.

A.B. Hill, 'Memories of the British Streptomycin Trial in Tuberculosis', *Controlled Clinical Trials*, 11 (1990), 77–9.

A.B. Hill, *Principles of Medical Statistics*, 1st edn (London: *Lancet*, 1937).

A.B. Hill, *Principles of Medical Statistics*, 2nd edn (London: *Lancet*, 1939).

A.B. Hill, *Principles of Medical Statistics*, 3rd edn (London: *Lancet*, 1942).

A.B. Hill, *Principles of Medical Statistics*, 4th edn (London: *Lancet*, 1948).

A.B. Hill, *Principles of Medical Statistics*, 5th edn (London: *Lancet*, 1952).

A.B. Hill, *Principles of Medical Statistics*, 6th edn (London: *Lancet*, 1955).

A.B. Hill, *The Start and Early Years of my Career* (Manuscript collection of the London School of Hygiene and Tropical Medicine, 1988).

G.B. Hill, 'Controlled Clinical Trials: The Emergence of a Paradigm', *Clinical and Investigative Medicine*, 6 (1983), 25–32.

L. Hill, 'Effects of Ultra-Violet Radiation', *British Medical Journal*, i (1926), 617–18.

Bibliography

L. Hill, 'Influence of Sunlight and Artificial Light on Health', *British Medical Journal,* ii (1925), 470–3.

T.J. Hollins, 'Treatment of Diabetes by Raw Fresh Gland (Pancreas)', *British Medical Journal,* i (1925), 503–4.

T.J. Hollins, 'Treatment of Diabetes by Raw Fresh Gland (Pancreas)', *British Medical Journal,* i (1925), 946–7.

T. Horder, *Health and a Day* (London: J.M. Dent, 1937).

R. Hutchinson, 'Fashions and Fads in Medicine', *British Medical Journal,* i (1925), 995–8.

A. Innes, 'Insulin Treatment Without Blood Sugar Estimations', *British Medical Journal,* i (1924), 55–6.

M. Kenney *et al.*, 'p-aminobenzenesulphonamide in Treatment of Bacterium Coli Infections of the Urinary Tract', *Lancet,* ii (1937), 119–25.

J. King, 'Ultra-Violet Rays in Medicine', *British Medical Journal,* ii (1930), 975.

R. King-Brown, 'Artificial Light Treatment', *The Times,* 16 March 1929.

R. King-Brown, 'Conference on "Light and Heat in Medicine"', *British Medical Journal,* ii (1927), 1194.

R. King-Brown, 'A Critical Review of the Colebrook Report in Irradiation of School Children', *British Journal of Actinotherapy and Physiotherapy,* 4 (1929), 168–70.

W. Langdon Brown, 'Endocrine Therapy', *Lancet,* i (1925), 739.

R.D. Lawrence, *The Diabetic Life: Its Control by Diet and Insulin* (London: J. & A. Churchill, 1925), 10.

R.D. Lawrence, 'Raw Pancreas by Mouth Compared with Insulin', *British Medical Journal,* i (1925), 1108.

R.D. Lawrence, 'Raw Pancreas by Mouth Compared with Insulin', *British Medical Journal,* ii (1925), 920.

R.D. Lawrence, 'Raw Pancreas by the Mouth in the Treatment of Diabetes', *British Medical Journal,* ii (1925), 87.

T. Lewis, 'Research in Medicine: Its Position and Needs', *British Medical Journal,* i (1930), 479–83.

J.P. Lockhart-Mummery, 'The Royal Society Discussion on "Experimental Production of Malignant Tumours"', *Lancet,* ii (1933), 323.

W.R. Logan and J.T. Smeall, 'A Direct Method of Typing Pneumococci', *British Medical Journal,* i (1932), 188–9.

W.R. Logan and J.T. Smeall, 'Direct Pneumococcal Typing', *British Medical Journal,* i (1932), 305–6.

J. Lynn-Thomas, 'Artificial Light: Treatment of Rickets', *The Times,* 20 March 1929, 12.

D.M. Lyon and W.L. Lamb, 'Difficulties in Comparing Methods of Treatment for Lobar Pneumonia', *Edinburgh Medical Journal,* 36 (1929), 79–93.

I.M. Macintyre, 'Tribulations for Clinical Trials', *British Medical Journal,* 302 (1991), 1099–100.

H.M. Mackay, 'Artificial Light Therapy in Infancy', *Archives of Disease in Childhood,* 2 (1927), 231–46.

R.L. Mackenzie Wallis, 'The Internal Secretion of the Pancreas and its Application to the Treatment of Diabetes Mellitus', *Lancet,* ii (1922), 1158–61.

H. Maclean and R.D. Lawrence, 'Oral Administration of Pancreatic Preparations in the Treatment of Diabetes', *British Medical Journal,* ii (1926), 323–4.

J.J.R. Macleod, 'Insulin and Diabetes', *British Medical Journal,* ii (1922), 833–5.

J.S. Maxwell, 'The Treatment of Post-Operative Retention of Urine with "Doryl"', *Lancet,* i (1937), 263–4.

J. McCormack and T. Greenhalgh, 'Seeing What You Want to See in Randomised Controlled Trials: Versions and Perversions of UKPDS Data', *British Medical Journal,* 320 (2000), 1720–3.

I.R. McEwen, 'Case Reports: Slices of Real Life to Complement Evidence', *Physical Therapy,* 84 (2004), 126–7.

Medical Directory (London: John Churchill and Sons, 1925).

Medical Research Council, 'Clinical Trials of New Remedies', *Lancet,* ii (1931), 304.

Medical Research Council, 'Clinical Trials of Influenza Vaccine', *British Medical Journal,* ii (1953), 1173–7.

Medical Research Council, *Report of the Medical Research Council for the Year 1927–1928* (London: HMSO, 1929).

Medical Research Council, *Report of the Medical Research Council for the Year 1930–1931* (London: HMSO, 1932).

Bibliography

Medical Research Council, *Report of the Medical Research Council for the Year 1932–1933* (London: HMSO, 1934).

Medical Research Council, *Report of the Medical Research Council for the Year 1933–1934* (London: HMSO, 1935).

Medical Research Council, *Report of the Medical Research Council for the Year 1934–1935* (London: HMSO, 1936).

Medical Research Council, *Report of the Medical Research Council for the Year 1935–1936* (London: HMSO, 1937).

Medical Research Council, *Report of the Medical Research Council for the Year 1936–1937* (London: HMSO, 1938).

Medical Research Council, *Report of the Medical Research Council for the Year 1937–1938* (London: HMSO, 1939).

Medical Research Council, *Report of the Medical Research Council for the Year 1938–1939* (London: HMSO, 1940).

Medical Research Council, *Report of the Medical Research Council for the Years 1945–1948* (London: HMSO, 1949).

Medical Research Council, 'Report to the Medical Research Council: Insulin and the Treatment of Diabetes: Some Clinical Results', *Lancet*, i (1923), 905–8.

Medical Research Council Streptomycin in Tuberculosis Trials Committee, 'Streptomycin Treatment for Pulmonary Tuberculosis', *British Medical Journal*, ii (1948), 769–82.

Medical Research Council, Therapeutic Trials Committee of the, 'The Serum Treatment of Lobar Pneumonia', *British Medical Journal*, i (1934), 241–5.

Medical Who's Who, 7th edn (London: The London & Counties Press Association Ltd, 1925).

H. Mellanby *et al.*, 'Vaccination against Influenza A', *Lancet*, 1 (1948), 978–82.

G.H.S. Milln, 'Ultra-Violet Ray Therapy', *British Medical Journal*, i (1927), 567.

C. Moir, 'The Use of "Doryl" (Carbaminoyl-choline) in Post-Operative and Post-Partum Retention of Urine', *Lancet*, i (1937), 261–3.

S. Moore, 'Artificial Sunlight Treatment of Feeble Children', *British Medical Journal*, ii (1927), 468.

W. Moore, 'Faith Healing', *The Observer*, 15 December 2002.

B. Moynihan, 'The Relation of Medicine to the Natural Sciences', *Lancet*, i (1925),115–7, 117;), 209.

Bibliography

G. Murray Levick, 'Artificial Light Therapy', *The Times,* 18 March 1929.

G. Murray Levick, 'The Therapeutic Value of Ultra-Violet Light', *British Medical Journal,* i (1929), 620.

A. Ness, S.J. Frankel, D.J. Gunnell, and G. Davey Smith, 'Are We Really Dying for a Tan?', *British Medical Journal,* 319 (1999), 114–16.

E.F. Neve, 'Raw Pancreas in Diabetes Mellitus', *British Medical Journal,* i (1926), 476.

J.A. Nixon, 'Diabetes and Insulin', *British Medical Journal,* i (1924), 53–5.

R.A. O'Brien, 'The Treatment of Pneumonia', *British Medical Journal,* i (1931), 446–8.

R.A. O'Brien, 'Specific Serum Treatment of Lobar Pneumonia in Adults', *British Medical Journal,* i (1931), 557–8.

W.H. Park, J.G. Bullowa and M.B. Rosenbluth, 'The Treatment of Lobar Pneumonia with Refined Specific Antibacterial Serum', *Journal of the American Medical Association,* 91, 29 (1928), 1503–8.

G.F. Petrie, 'Specific Serum Treatment of Lobar Pneumonia in Adults', *British Medical Journal,* i (1931), 557.

A. Physician, 'Some Thoughts about Endocrinology', *Lancet,* i (1923), 207.

H. Pomeroy Kelly, 'Treatment of Diabetes by Raw Fresh Gland (Pancreas)', *British Medical Journal,* i (1925), 921.1

F.W. Price, *A Textbook of the Practice of Medicine* (Fourth Edition, London: H. Milford, Oxford University Press, 1933), 22.

E. Richards, *Vitamin C and Cancer: Medicine or Politics?* (Basingstoke: Macmillan, 1991).

P.F. Ridgway and A.W. Darzi, 'Placebos and Standardising New Surgical Techniques', *British Medical Journal,* 325 (2002), 560.

A. Roberts, 'Ultra-Violet Light from Open Arc with Titanium Electrodes', *British Medical Journal,* i (1927), 184–6.

R. Robertson Young, 'Treatment of Diabetes by Raw Fresh Gland (Pancreas)', *British Medical Journal,* i (1925), 632.

J. Russell, 'Could These Foods be Giving Us Cancer?' *The Guardian,* 15 August 2002.

I. Russell, 'Evaluating New Surgical Procedures', *British Medical Journal,* 311 (1995), 1243–4.

Bibliography

J.A. Ryle, 'Serum Treatment of Pneumonia', *British Medical Journal,* ii (1932), 263.

G.B. Shaw, 'Sir Almroth Wright', *British Medical Journal,* i (1947), 659.

A. Sheikh, L. Smeeth and R. Ashcroft, 'Randomised Controlled Trials in Primary Care: Scope and Application', *British Journal, of General Practice,* 52 (2002), 746–51.

A.H. Smith, 'Concentrated Antipneumococcal Serum in the Treatment of Lobar Pneumonia', *British Medical Journal,* i (1931), 818.

W. Smith, C. Andrewes and P. Laidlaw, 'A Virus Obtained from Influenza Patients', *Lancet,* 2 (1933), 66–8.

R. Smith, 'Babies and Consent: Yet Another NHS Scandal', *British Medical Journal,* 320 (2000), 1285–6.

W.R. Snodgrass and T. Anderson, 'Prontosil in the Treatment of Erysipelas: A Controlled Series of 312 Cases', *British Medical Journal,* ii (1937), 101–4.

W.R. Snodgrass and T. Anderson, 'Sulphanilamide in the Treatment of Erysipelas: A Controlled Series of 270 Cases', *British Medical Journal,* ii (1937), 1156–9.

J.C. Spence, 'Clinical Tests of the Antirachitic Activity of Calciferol', *Lancet,* ii (1933), 911–5.

C.H. Stuart-Harris, 'Influenza Epidemics and the Influenza Viruses', *British Medical Journal,* i (1945), 251–7.

C.H. Stuart-Harris, W. Smith and C.H. Andrewes, 'The Influenza Epidemic of January- March, 1939', *British Medical Journal,* i (1940), 205–11.

M.D. Sullivan, 'Placebo Controls and Epistemic Control in Orthodox Medicine', *Journal of Medical Philosophy,* 18, 2 (1993), 213–31.

A.G. Sutcliffe, 'Prescribing Medicines for Children', *British Medical Journal,* 319 (1999), 70–1.

F. Theobalds, 'Polyglandular Therapy', *British Medical Journal,* ii (1923), 209.

J. Tonking, 'Individual Overdose of Ultra-Violet Rays', *British Medical Journal,* i (1926), 462.

D. Torgerson and B. Sibbald, 'Understanding Controlled Trials: What is a Patient Preference Trial?', *British Medical Journal,* 316 (1998), 360.

U.S. Influenza Commission, 'The U.S. Influenza Commission', *Journal of the American Medical Association* 124 (1944), 982.

D. Van der Windt B.W. Koes, M. Van Aarst, M.A. Heemskerk, and L.M. Bouter, 'Practical Aspects of Conducting a Pragmatic Randomised Trial in Primary Care: Patient Recruitment and Outcome Assessment', *British Journal of General Practice,* 50 (2000), 371–4.

S. Vincent, 'The Present Position of Organotherapy', *Lancet,* i (1923), 130–32.

S. Vincent, 'The Uses and Abuses of Endocrine Therapy', *Lancet,* ii (1925), 331–2.

E.J. Wayne, 'Clinical Observations on Two Pure Glucosides of Digitalis, Digoxin and Digitalinum Verum', *Clinical Science,* 1 (1933), 63–76.

M. Weinbren, 'Varicose Ulcers: Ultra-Violet Light and Unna's Paste Dressings', *Lancet,* i (1928), 1302.

M. Weinbren, 'The Uses of Ultra-Violet Light', *Lancet,* i (1929), 685.

J. Wells, 'Mammography and the Politics of Randomised Controlled Trials', *British Medical Journal,* 317 (1998), 1224–30.

A.J. Welton, M.R. Vickers, J.A. Cooper, T.W. Meade, and T.M. Marteau, 'Is Recruitment More Difficult with a Placebo Arm in Randomised Controlled Trials? A Quasirandomised, Interview Based Study', *British Medical Journal,* 318 (1999), 1114–7.

J.F. Wilkinson and M.C.G. Israels, 'The Pentnucleotide Treatment of Agranulocytic Angina', *Lancet,* ii (1934), 353–5.

J.F. Wilkinson, 'The Value of Extracts of Suprarenal Cortex in the Treatment of Addison's Disease', *Lancet,* ii (1937), 61–70.

T.O. Williams, 'More Blasts on the Trumpet', *British Medical Journal,* ii (1951), 1218.

A.E. Wright, 'An Address on Wound Infections: And on some Methods for the Study of the Various Factors which Come into Consideration in their Treatment', in A.E. Wright, *Pathology and Treatment of War Wounds* (London: Heinemann, 1942), 1–29.

A.E. Wright, 'On the Possible Advantages of Employing Decalcified Milk in the Feeding of Infants and Invalids', *Lancet,* ii (1893), 194.

A.E. Wright, *The Unexpurgated Case Against Woman's Suffrage* (London: Constable, 1913).

A.E. Wright, 'On Vaccine Therapy and Immunisation in Vitro', *Lancet,* ii (1931), 225–30.

Bibliography

A.E. Wright (ed.), *Vaccine Therapy, its Administration, Value and Limitations: A Discussion Opened by Sir Almroth E. Wright* (London: Longmans, Green & Co., 1910).

Secondary sources

E.H. Ackerknecht, *Therapeutics from the Primitives to the Twentieth Century* (New York: Hafner Press, 1973).

L.K. Altman, *Who Goes First? The Story of Self-Experimentation in Medicine.* (Berkeley: University of California Press, 1998).

O. Amsterdamska, 'Chemistry in the Clinic: The Research Career of Donald Dexter van Slyke', in S. de Chadarevian and H. Kamminga (eds.), *Molecularizing Biology: New Practices and Alliances, 1910s–1970s* (Amsterdam: OPA, 1998).

D. Armstrong, 'Clinical Autonomy, Individual and Collective: The Problem of Changing Doctors' Behaviour', *Social Science and Medicine,* 55 (2002), 1771–7.

H. Atkins, 'Conduct of a Controlled Clinical Trial', *British Medical Journal* , 2 (1966), 377–9.

J. Austoker, *A History of the Imperial Cancer Research Fund 1902–1986* (Oxford: Oxford University Press, 1988).

J. Austoker and L. Bryder, 'The National Institute for Medical Research and Related Activities of the MRC', in J. Austoker and L. Bryder (eds), *Historical Perspectives on the role of the MRC.* (Oxford: Oxford University Press, 1989), 35–57.

J. Austoker, 'Walter Morley Fletcher and the Origins of a Basic Biomedical Research Policy', in J. Austoker and L. Bryder (eds), *Historical Perspectives on the Role of the MRC.* (Oxford: Oxford University Press, 1989), 23–33.

C. Bazerman, *Shaping Written Knowledge: The Genre and Activity of the Experimental Article in Science* (Madison: University of Wisconsin Press, 1988).

S. Bennett, 'The Industrial Instrument: Master of Industry, Servant of Management: Automatic Control in the Process Industries, 1900–1940', *Technology and Culture* 32, 1 (1991), 69–81.

W.I.B. Beveridge, *Influenza: The Last Great Plague* (London: Heinemann, 1977).

Bibliography

G.G.L. Biondi-Zoccai, M. Lotrionte, A. Abbate, L. Testa, E. Remigi, F. Burzotta, M. Valgimigli, E. Romagnoli, F. Crea, P. Agostoni, 'Compliance with QUOROM and Quality of Reporting of Overlapping Meta-Analyses on the Role of Acetylcysteine in the Prevention of Contrast Associated Nephropathy: Case Study', *British Medical Journal*, 332 (2006), 202–6.

M. Borell, 'Setting the Standards for a New Science: Edward Schafer and Endocrinology', *Medical History*, 22 (1978), 282–90.

E.G. Boring, 'The Nature and History of Experimental Control', *American Journal of Psychology*, 67 (1954), 573–89.

A.M. Brandt and M. Gardner, 'The Golden Age of Medicine?' in R. Cooter and J. Pickstone (eds), *Medicine in the Twentieth Century* (Amsterdam: Harwood, 2000), 21–37.

J.P. Bull, 'The Historical Development of Clinical Therapeutic Trials', *Journal of Chronic Diseases,* 10 (1959), 218–48.

D. Cantor, 'The MRC's Support for Experimental Radiology during the Inter-War Years', in J. Austoker and L. Bryder (eds), *Historical Perspectives on the Role of the MRC* (Oxford: Oxford University Press, 1989), 181–204.

C. Ceballos, J.R. Valdizan, A. Artal, C. Almarcegui, C. Allepuz, J. Garcia Campayo, R. Fernandez Liesa, P. Giraldo, and T. Puertolas, 'Why Evidence-Based Medicine? 20 Years of Meta-Analysis', *Anales de Medicina Interna*, 17, 10 (2000), 521–6. (Spanish article, English abstract).

I. Chalmers, 'Comparing Like with Like: Some Historical Milestones in the Evolution of Methods to Create Unbiased Comparison Groups in Therapeutic Experiments', *International Journal of Epidemiology*, 30 (2001), 1156–64.

I. Chalmers, 'MRC Therapeutic Trials Committee's Report on Serum Treatment of Lobar Pneumonia, BMJ 1934', in The James Lind library (www.jameslindlibrary.org) accessed 4 July 2007.

I. Chalmers, 'Statistical Theory was not the Reason that Randomization was used in the British Medical Research Council's Clinical Trial of Streptomycin for Pulmonary Tuberculosis', in G. Jorland, A. Opinel and G. Weisz (eds), *Body Counts: Medical Quantification in Historical and Sociological Perspectives* (Montreal: McGill-Queen's University Press, 2005), 309–34.

I. Chalmers, 'Unbiased, Relevant, and Reliable Assessments in Health Care', *British Medical Journal,* 317 (1998), 1167–8.

Bibliography

I. Chalmers, C. Rounding and K. Lock, 'Descriptive Survey of Non-Commercial Randomised Controlled Trials in the United Kingdom, 1980–2002', *British Medical Journal,* 327 (2003), 1017–20.

A. Chase, *Magic shots: A Human and Scientific Account of the Long and Continuing Struggle to Eradicate Infectious Diseases by Vaccination* (New York: Morrow, 1982).

W. Coleman, *Biology in the Nineteenth Century: Problems of Form, Function, and Transformation* (Cambridge: Cambridge University Press, 1977).

R. Collins R. Peto, R. Gray and S. Parish, 'Large-Scale Randomized Evidence: Trials and Overviews', in D. Warrell, T.M. Cox, J.D. Firth, E.J. Benz, and D. Weatherall (eds), *Oxford Textbook of Medicine, Volume 1,* 4th edn (Oxford: Oxford University Press, 2003), 24–36.

D.C.T Cox-Maksimov, *The Making of the Clinical Trial in Britain, 1910–1945: Expertise, The State and the Public* (PhD thesis: Cambridge University, 1998).

J. Daly, *Evidence-Based Medicine and the Search for a Science of Clinical Care* (Berkeley: University of California Press, 2005).

T. Dehue, 'Deception, Efficiency, and Random Groups: Psychology and the Gradual Origination of the Random Group Design', *Isis,* 88, 4 (1997), 653–73.

T. Dehue, 'From Deception Trials to Control Reagents: The Introduction of the Control Group about a Century Ago', *American Psychologist,* 55, 2 (2000), 264–8.

N. Demand, 'Did the Greeks Believe in the Efficacy of Hippocratic Treatment – and, if so, Why?' in I. Garofalo, A. Lami, D. Manetti, and A. Roselli (eds), *Aspetti della Terapia nel Corpus Hippocraticum* (Florence: Olschki, 1999).

A. Digby and N. Bosanquet, 'Doctors and Patients in an Era of National Health Insurance and Private Practice, 1913-1938', *Economic History Review,* 2nd ser., XLI , 1 (1988), 74–94.

R. Doll, 'Controlled Trials: The 1948 Watershed', *British Medical Journal,* 317 (1998), 1217–20.

M. Dunnill, *The Plato of Praed Street: The Life and Times of Almroth Wright* (London: Royal Society of Medicine Press, 2000), 240.

E. Ebstein, 'Medical Men who Experimented upon Themselves', *Medical Life,* 38 (1931), 216–18.

Bibliography

S.J.L. Edwards, R.J. Lilford and J. Hewison, 'The Ethics of Randomised Controlled Trials from the Perspectives of Patients, the Public. and Healthcare Professionals', *British Medical Journal,* 317 (1998), 1209–12.

S. Epstein, *Impure Science: AIDS, Activism, and the Politics of Knowledge* (Berkeley: University of California Press, 1996).

C. Feudtner, *Bittersweet: Diabetes, Insulin and the Transformation of Illness* (Chapel Hill: University of North Carolina Press, 2003).

D. Fisher, 'The Rockefeller Foundation and the Development of Scientific Medicine in Great Britain', *Minerva,* XVI (1978), 21–41.

L. Fitzgerald and S. Dopson, 'Knowledge, Credible Evidence, and Utilization', in S. Dopson and L. Fitzgerald (eds.), *Knowledge to Action? Evidence-Based Health Care in Context* (Oxford: Oxford University Press, 2005), 132–54.

M. Fletcher, *The Bright Countenance: A Personal Biography of Walter Morley Fletcher* (London: Hodder and Stoughton, 1957).

A.C. Freeman and K. Sweeney, 'Why General Practitioners Do Not Implement Evidence: Qualitative Study', *British Medical Journal,* 323 (2001), 1100–2.

G.L. Geison, 'Divided we Stand: Physiologists and Clinicians in the American Context', in M. Vogel and C. Rosenberg (eds), *The Therapeutic Revolution: Essays in the Social History of American Medicine* (Pennsylvania: University of Pennsylvania Press, 1979), 67–90.

J. Golinski, *Making Natural Knowledge: Constructivism and the History of Science* (Cambridge: Cambridge University Press, 1998).

J. Goodman, 'Pharmaceutical Industry', in R. Cooter and J. Pickstone (eds), *Medicine in the Twentieth Century* (Amsterdam: Harwood, 2000), 141–54.

G. Graham, 'The Formation of the Medical and Surgical Professorial Units in the London Teaching Hospitals', *Annals of Science,* 26 (1970), 1–22.

T. Greenhalgh, 'Intuition and Evidence: Uneasy Bedfellows?', *British Journal of General Practice* 52 (2002), 395–400.

T. Greenhalgh and B. Hurwitz, 'Narrative Based Medicine: Why Study Narrative?' *British Medical Journal,* 318 (1999), 48–50.

I. Hacking, 'Telepathy: Origins of Randomization in Experimental Design', *Isis,* 79 (1988), 427–51.

E. Higgs, 'Medical Statistics, Patronage and the State: The Development of the MRC Statistical Unit, 1911–1948', *Medical History,* 44 (2000), 323–40.

Bibliography

D. Holmes, S.J. Murray, A. Perron and G. Rail, 'Deconstructing the Evidence-Based Discourse in Health Sciences: Truth, Power and Fascism', *International Journal of Evidence-Based Healthcare,* 4, 3 (2006), 180–6.

A.R. Jadad, M. Moher, G.P. Browman, L. Booker, C. Sigouin, M. Fuentes, and R. Stevens, 'Systematic Reviews and Meta-Analyses on Treatment of Asthma: Critical Evaluation', *British Medical Journal,* 320 (2000), 537–40.

T. Kaptchuk, 'Intentional Ignorance: A History of Blind Assessment and Placebo Controls', *Bulletin of the History of Medicine,* 72 (1998), 389–433.

P. Kitcher, 'Persuasion', in M. Pera and W. Shea (eds), *Persuading Science: The Art of Scientific Rhetoric* (Canton: Science History Publications, 1991), 3–27.

G.J. Kutcher, *Clinical Ethics and Research Imperatives in Human Experiments: A Case of Contested Knowledge* (PhD thesis: Cambridge University, 2001).

G. Lakoff and M. Johnson, *Metaphors We Live By* (Chicago: University of Chicago Press, 1980).

A. Landsborough Thomson, *Half a Century of Medical Research. Volume One: Origins and Policy of the Medical Research Council (UK)* (London: HMSO, 1973).

A. Landsborough Thomson, *Half a Century of Medical Research. Volume Two: The Programme of the Medical Research Council (UK)* (London: Medical Research Council, 1987).

C. Langford, 'The Age Pattern of Mortality in the 1918-19 Influenza Pandemic: An Attempted Explanation Based on Data for England and Wales', *Medical History,* 46 (2002), 1–20.

C. Lawrence, 'Clinical Research', in J. Krige and D. Pestre (eds), *Science in the Twentieth Century.* (Amsterdam: Harwood, 1997), 439–59.

C. Lawrence, 'Incommunicable Knowledge: Science, Technology and the Clinical Art in Britain 1850–1914', *Journal of Contemporary History,* 20 (1985), 503–20.

C. Lawrence, *Medicine in the Making of Modern Britain 1700–1920* (London: Routledge, 1994), 72–6.

C. Lawrence, *Rockefeller Money, the Laboratory, and Medicine in Edinburgh 1919–1930: New Science in an Old Country* (Rochester, New York: University of Rochester Press, 2005).

C. Lawrence and R. Dixey, 'Practising on Principle: Joseph Lister and the Germ Theories of Disease', in C. Lawrence (ed.), *Medical Theory, Surgical Practice: Studies in the History of Surgery* (London: Routledge, 1992), 153–215.

206

Bibliography

G. Lawrence, 'Tools of the Trade: The Finsen Light', *Lancet,* 359 (2002), 1784.

J. Liebenau, 'The MRC and the Pharmaceutical Industry: The Model of Insulin', in J. Austoker and L. Bryder (eds), *Historical Perspectives on the Role of the MRC* (Oxford: Oxford University Press, 1989), 163–80.

A.M. Lilienfeld, 'Ceteris Paribus: The Evolution of the Clinical Trial', *Bulletin of the History of Medicine,* 56 (1982), 1–18.

S. Lock, 'The Randomised Controlled Trial: A British Invention', in G. Lawrence (ed.), *Technologies of Modern Medicine* (London: The Science Museum, 1994), 81–7.

D. Long Hall, 'The Critic and the Advocate: Contrasting British Views on the State of Endocrinology in the Early 1920s', *Journal of the History of Biology,* 2 (1976), 269–85.

I. Lowy, *Between Bench and Bedside: Science, Healing and Interleukin-2 in a Cancer Ward* (Cambridge: Harvard University Press, 1996).

A. Maehle, *Drugs on Trial: Experimental Pharmacology and Therapeutic Innovation in the Eighteenth Century* (Amsterdam: Rodopi, 1999).

H.M. Marks, 'Notes from the Underground: The Social Organization of Therapeutic Research', in R.C. Maulitz and D.E. Long (eds), *Grand Rounds: One Hundred Years of Internal Medicine* (Philadelphia: University of Pennsylvania Press, 1988), 297–336.

H.M. Marks, *The Progress of Experiment: Science and Therapeutic Reform in the United States, 1900–1990* (Cambridge: Cambridge University Press, 1997).

J.R. Matthews, *Quantification and the Quest for Medical Certainty* (Princeton: Princeton University Press, 1995).

R.C. Maulitz, '"Physician versus Bacteriologist": The Ideology of Science in Clinical Medicine', in M. Vogel and C. Rosenberg (eds), *The Therapeutic Revolution: Essays in the Social History of American Medicine* (Pennsylvania: University of Pennsylvania Press, 1979), 91–107.

M. Meldrum, *"Departures from Design": The Randomized Clinical Trial in Historical Context, 1946–1970* (PhD thesis: State University of New York at Stony Brook, 1994).

S.L. Montgomery, *The Scientific Voice* (New York: Guilford Press, 1996).

E.T. Morman (ed.), *Efficiency, Scientific Management and Hospital Standardization: An Anthology of Sources* (New York: Garland, 1989).

Bibliography

M. Nothman, 'The History of the Discovery of Pancreatic Diabetes', *Bulletin of the History of Medicine*, XXVIII (1954), 272–4.

S.F. Olsen, 'Use of Randomisation in Early Clinical Trials', *British Medical Journal*, 318 (1999), 1352.

J. Parascandola, 'The Search for the Active Oxytocic Principle of Ergot: Laboratory Science and Clinical Medicine in Conflict', in E. Hickel and G. Schröder (eds), *Neue Beiträge zur Arzneimittelgeschichte*, Vol. 51 of *Veröffentlichungen der Internationalen Gesellschaft för Geschichte der Pharmazie e. V.* (Stuttgart: Wissenschaftliche Verlagsgesellschaft, 1982), 205–27.

H.J. Parish, *Victory with Vaccines: The Story of Immunization* (Edinburgh: E & S Livingstone, 1968).

M. Pera, 'The Role and Value of Rhetoric in Science', in M. Pera and W. Shea (eds), *Persuading Science: The Art of Scientific Rhetoric* (Canton: Science History Publications, 1991), 29–54.

R. Peto and C. Baigent, 'Trials: The Next Fifty Years', *British Medical Journal*, 317 (1998), 1170–1.

S.J. Pocock, 'The Historical Development of Clinical Trials', in S.J. Pocock, *Clinical Trials: A Practical Approach* (Chichester: John Wiley, 1983), 14–27.

T.M. Porter, *Trust in Numbers: Objectivity in Science and Public Life* (Princeton: Princeton University Press, 1995).

G. Risse, 'The History of Therapeutics', in W.F. Bynum and V. Nutton (eds), *Essays in the History of Therapeutics* (Amsterdam: Rodopi, 1991), 3–11.

C.E. Rosenberg, 'The Therapeutic Revolution: Medicine, Meaning, and Social Change in Nineteenth-Century America', in M.J. Vogel and C.E. Rosenberg (eds), *The Therapeutic Revolution: Essays in the Social History of American Medicine* (Pennsylvania: University of Pennsylvania Press, 1979), 3–25.

S. Schaffer, 'Self Evidence', *Critical Inquiry*, 18 (1992), 327–62.

J. Schuster and R. Yeo, 'Introduction', in J. Schuster and R. Yeo (eds), *The Politics and Rhetoric of Scientific Method* (Dordecht & Boston: Kluwer, 1986), ix–xxxvii.

J. Scott and G. Marshall, 'Scientific Management', in *A Dictionary of Sociology*, *Oxford Reference Online* (Oxford: Oxford University Press, 2005).

S. Shapere, 'On Deciding what to Believe and how to Talk about Nature', in M. Pera and W. Shea (eds.), *Persuading Science: The Art of Scientific Rhetoric* (Canton: Science History Publications, 1991), 89–103.

Bibliography

S. Shapin, *A Social History of Truth: Civility and Science in Seventeenth-Century England.* (Chicago: University of Chicago Press, 1994).

A.K. Shapiro and E. Shapiro, *The Powerful Placebo: From Ancient Priest to Modern Physician* (Baltimore: Johns Hopkins University Press, 1997).

R. Smith, 'Fifty Years of Randomised Controlled Trials', *British Medical Journal,* 317 (1998), 7167.

R. Smith, *Inhibition: History and Meaning in the Sciences of Mind and Brain* (London: Free Association Books, 1992).

R. Stevens, *Medical Practice in Modern England* (New Haven: Yale University Press, 1966).

S. Sturdy, 'From the Trenches to the Hospitals at Home: Physiologists, Clinicians and Oxygen Therapy, 1914–30', in J. Pickstone (ed.), *Medical Innovations in Historical Perspective* (Basingstoke: Palgrave MacMillan, 1992), 104–23.

S. Sturdy and R. Cooter, 'Science, Scientific Management, and the Transformation of Medicine in Britain c. 1870–1950', *History of Science*, 34, 4 (1998), 421–66.

K. Sweeney, 'Personal Knowledge', *British Medical Journal* 332 (2006), 129–30.

R.B. Tattersall, 'A Force of Magical Activity: The Introduction of Insulin Treatment in Britain 1922–1926', *Diabetic Medicine* 12 (1995), 730–55.

R.B. Tattersall, 'Pancreatic Organotherapy for Diabetes 1889-1921', *Medical History,* 39 (1995), 288–316,

R.B. Tattersall, 'The Quest for Normoglycaemia: A Historical Perspective', *Diabetic Medicine,* 11 (1994), 618–35.

S. Timmermans and M. Berg, *The Gold Standard: The Challenge of Evidence-Based Medicine and Standardization in Health Care* (Philadelphia: Temple University Press, 2003).

B. Toth, *Clinical Trials in British Medicine 1858–1948, with Special Reference to the Development of the Randomised Controlled Trial* (PhD thesis: University of Bristol, 1998).

U. Tröhler, *'To Improve the Evidence of Medicine': The Eighteenth Century British Origins of a Critical Approach* (Edinburgh: Royal College of Physicians of Edinburgh, 2000).

K. Wailoo, *Drawing Blood: Technology and Disease Identity in Twentieth Century America* (Baltimore: Johns Hopkins University Press, 1997).

Bibliography

J.H. Warner, *The Therapeutic Perspective: Medical Practice, Knowledge and Identity in America, 1820–1885* (Princeton: Princeton University Press, 1997)

P. Weindling, 'From Medical Research to Clinical Practice: Serum Therapy for Diphtheria in the 1890s', in J. Pickstone (ed.), *Medical Innovations in Historical Perspective* (Basingstoke: Macmillan, 1992), 72–83.

G. Weisz, 'From Clinical Counting to Evidence-Based Medicine', in G. Jorland, A. Opinel and G. Weisz (eds), *Body Counts: Medical Quantification in Historical and Sociological Perspective* (Montreal: McGill-Queen's University Press, 2005), 377–93.

L.A. Whaley, *Women's History as Scientists: A Guide to the Debates* (Santa Barbara, California: ABC-Clio, 2003).

R. Williams, *Keywords* (London: Fontana, 1988).

M. Worboys, 'Vaccine Therapy and Laboratory Medicine in Edwardian Britain', in J. Pickstone (ed.), *Medical Innovations in Historical Perspective* (Basingstoke: Macmillan, 1992), 84–103.

R. Yeo, 'Scientific Method and the Rhetoric of Science in Britain, 1830–1917', in J. Schuster and R. Yeo (eds), *The Politics and Rhetoric of Scientific Method* (Dordecht & Boston: Kluwer, 1986), 259–97.

A.Y. Yoshioka, *Streptomycin, 1946: British Central Administration of Supplies of a New Drug of American Origin with Special Reference to Clinical Trials in Tuberculosis* (PhD thesis: Imperial College, University of London, 1998).

R. Young, *Darwin's Metaphor: Nature's Place in Victorian Culture* (Cambridge, England: Cambridge University Press, 1985).

Index

A

Printed in the United States
by Baker & Taylor Publisher Services